Pediatric
Clinical Problem Solving

Pediatric
Clinical Problem Solving

Vincent A. Fulginiti, M.D.

Professor and Head
Department of Pediatrics
Arizona Health Sciences Center
Tucson, Arizona

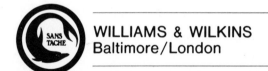

WILLIAMS & WILKINS
Baltimore/London

Made in the United States of America

Library of Congress Cataloging in Publication Data

Fulginiti, Vincent A.
  Pediatric clinical problem solving.

  Bibliography: p.
    1. Pediatrics—Problems, exercises, etc. 2. Pediatrics—Case studies. 3. Pediatrics—Decision making. 4. Medical logic. 5. Problem solving. I. Title. [DNLM: 1. Pediatrics. 2. Problem solving. WS 200 F963p]
RJ48.2.F84   618.92'00076   81-926
ISBN 0-683-03383-2   AACR2

Composed and printed at the
Waverly Press, Inc.
Mt. Royal and Guilford Aves.
Baltimore, MD 21202, U.S.A.

This book is written as a direct communication to students and residents of pediatrics.

It is about the major function of pediatric practice—the problem-solving process. The book grew out of a series of teaching exercises held at the bedside, and in conference with medical students and residents, during the past 16 years. At these conferences and rounds it became apparent that students rarely thought about or analyzed how and why they reached clinical conclusions. They learned facts, acquired skills and began the long process of development of diagnostic and therapeutic capabilities. Although they solved problems constantly, most often they were unaware of the process by which they did so.

My first sessions, in which we discussed the how and why of clinical problem solving, were puzzling and confusing to most students and residents. Even today at the beginning of each series I brace myself for the initial puzzlement. Soon, however, everyone "catches on" and eagerly participates, apparently delighted in the exploration of how they think.

Many students have asked for references so that they may explore these areas on their own. Because of these requests I surveyed as much of the available material as I could find. To my surprise and dismay, very little is written for student or resident use in this area. A few texts purport to deal with this process but really concentrate on differential diagnosis, not the same thing as problem solving, and do so on a "content" basis. That is, they focus upon the clinical facts and either ignore the process, give passing reference to it, or obscure its discussion with other material. I decided to codify the exercises that my students and I had engaged in and to add a broader discussion of what a physician does. In addition, adequate references to available materials are included for the student or resident who wishes to delve more deeply into any aspect of the subject. One method incorporated fully in this text—that of the case-problem approach—will assist the reader in practicing diagnostic reasoning. By working through each case before reading the discussion, the reader can then compare his thoughts with the author's. Patients derived from my own experience and those of my associates over the years are presented with an opportunity for the student to practice his skill. So that he has *some* standard for comparison, an analysis of each case is presented, not only a discussion of the facts but how and why they are used at that point in the analysis.

This text almost wrote itself, derived as it was from thousands of conversations with students and residents. It is literally a conversation with you, the reader. It is very much my own thinking, and therefore all of you will not agree with what I've said, with the emphasis given some areas, the lack elsewhere, with my values, or with my reasoning. That cannot be helped in a discipline which permits latitude of thought, expression of controversial and opposite opinions, and even arbitrary, dogmatic statements based on little else but the ego of the speaker. In fact, sections of this book will speak to such latitude of both opinion and action in medicine.

The text is divided into two sections. The first covers the theory of pediatric problem solving, and the second applies the process to specific areas.

In the theoretical section I have attempted to detail and dissect the clinical problem-solving process. It has been divided into essential elements, each of which is considered in elaborate detail.

In the practical section I have chosen many pediatric topics to display problem solving in action. The selection is purposeful. First, not all problems could possibly be covered. Second, those areas that occur repetitiously in everyday practice were selected. Third, some problems were chosen because they best illustrate specific features of the theory of problem solving.

I'm indebted to many silent contributors to this volume. First to my two major mentors during my own education: Dr. Waldo E. "Bill" Nelson, formerly Professor and Head of the Department of Pediatrics at Temple University (St. Christopher's Hospital) and currently in a most active retirement as Editor of the *Journal of Pediatrics*, among other activities; and Dr. C. Henry Kempe, formerly Professor and Head of the Department of Pediatrics, University of Colorado School of Medicine in Denver, and also actively retired both in virologic research and as head of the Battered Child Institute at the University of Colorado. Both men are leaders in medical education and thought. Their contribution to this book is in the form of precepts, concepts and behavior they modeled. From them derived the combination of science and humanity that should be evident in every physician and that is preached in this book. Without their sustained influence this book would never have been written.

A different form of influence derived from students and residents with whom I have been associated over the years. Apart from the direct contributions their words and analyses made to the content of this book, they provided and continue to provide that much maligned, but precious, entity, inspiration. It has often been said that a teacher learns by teaching. This certainly has been true in my own career, and this book reflects what little I've learned during my contacts with those anonymous beings, the students and residents at the Universities of Colorado and Arizona and at Temple University.

There have been many friends and colleagues who indirectly lent their help, and a few who did so consciously. Inadvertent help came from all of those who corrected me and who were able to point out the errors in my thinking or behavior over the years. Deliberate help came from Ray L. Helfer, M.D., Professor of Pediatrics at Michigan State University's College of Human Medicine. Throughout the entire process, Ray has helped me think through the concepts, checked my words and, in general, acted as a friend but severe critic.

My most persistent critic has been my wife, Shirley, who never permits laxity of phrase or idea. She also trims my ego so that the prose does not become too pontifical. In addition, by her skillful management of our four active children, John, Jeff, Laura and Paul, and their assorted friends, permitted some time to be donated to the actual writing. They contributed by respecting the time spent at the desk and by encouraging me with such comments as, "How much did you write today?", delivered in a properly supervisory voice. With their persistence the book simply had to be completed.

Enabling me to keep my deadlines were Theresa Collins, Donna Keller and Ellen Hankocy. Jo Anne Jenkins did a spectacular job in insuring that all typescript was legible, in the right form, and on time. Her efforts are particularly appreciated in enabling me to complete this book. Some of the writing was done during a leave from my office, so that their efforts were doubly appreciated, as they had other duties and responsibilities.

CONTENTS

CHAPTER 17
The Child with Gastrointestinal Bleeding

CHAPTER 18
The Child Who Fails to Thrive

CHAPTER 19
The Child with a Rash of Infectious Origin

CHAPTER 20
Detailed Analysis of a Single Child with Pharyngitis

Bibliography

Chapter 1

Clinical Problem Solving: Introduction—Getting the Point

" I never thought of that before."

This response has been typical in the small group sessions conducted with and for students and residents over the years. It usually is part of a dialogue in an example case discussion which flows something similar to this:

STUDENT: I think I want to get a CBC, urinalysis and chest X-ray.

ME: Why?

STUDENT: Pardon?

ME: Why do you want those laboratory analyses at this point in your thinking?

STUDENT: (Stammers slightly) Well, (pause) I need them. (Silence) I mean, they're part of the usual work-up—they're routine.

ME: Why?

STUDENT: Pardon? Oh, you mean why are they routine?

ME: Yes, and why do you want the values they'll give you?

STUDENT: Well, I never thought of that before.

It is precisely because of such dialogues with their repetitive inclusion of phrases meaning that the student or resident had a new insight into the clinical process that this book was written. Students and residents learn to do things, to acquire facts and to "think" without ever truly thinking about the processes involved. One memorable student, whom I'll call Percy, during a discussion similar to the one above, developed an increasingly disdainful expression on his face as student after student expressed perplexity at the questions I was asking. Finally it was Percy's turn to analyze a portion of the problem. He immediately launched into an excellent pathophysiologic discussion and concluded with his list of "next steps," as he termed them. Included were some elaborate and sophisticated diagnostic measures, each of which was associated with substantial risk to the patient. I began my critique of his analysis (or, rather, led him into analyzing his own thought pattern) when he interrupted and said, "I don't see the point of this. I told you what I thought was going on in this patient and these studies will answer the questions raised. Who cares what my reasons are, apart from those I already gave you?"

His was a seemingly bright and intelligent analysis. After all, he had correctly identified the pathophysiologic deficits and was simply testing his ideas. My response was, "The patient cares and so do you." I then went on and placed those diagnostic steps in their clinical perspective and indicated the risks to the patient. After a lengthy discussion occupying two sessions, and involving almost all of the students, Percy indicated that he finally got the point. He had learned pathophysiology exceptionally well. He had then learned both by example on his clerkships and by reading what was available in the way of diagnostic tests. He married the two in his discussion but never thought the entire process through. He simply was treating ideas and not their application to a living patient. His final comment was, "I never realized that someday I would be doing these things to people."

This anecdote serves as a total rationale for the writing and reading of this book. A clinician indeed "does things to people." He is not a theoretical physicist dealing in abstract symbolism and universes. He deals with single patients, one by one, who come to him because they are ill or because they wish to avoid illness; they present him with a real problem. The ideal physician does not reach into the firmament and pull an abstraction from the clouds onto his patient. Rather, he thinks about the patient's problem and judiciously attempts to diagnose and treat it.

Much has been said about the dehumanization of medical practice. Some is true, a great deal is overstated, and a little is totally inaccurate. The hand-holding phase of medicine prevalent prior to the 1940's was the result of many forces. The basic humanity of physicians, the onslaught and inevitability of diseases for which the doctor had no or little explanation and could only prescribe palliatives, the intense need for patient and relative alike to have someone who could guide them through their misery and grief, all combined to produce bedside medicine with a large measure of sympathetic psychotherapy. An image grew of the physician as a friend, a tireless worker and an occasional healer. Some of the imagery was larger than life. *Saturday Evening Post* cover paintings by Norman Rockwell captured the legendary features of the country family doctor. He was always depicted as kindly, warm and available. He became an American legend alongside the pilgrim, the pioneer, the farmer and many other stereotypes.

Along came the scientific era which swept medical practice off its feet. In short order the physician was converted from a bedside psychotherapist to an office pharmacotherapist. Gone was the impotence of ignorance and a pharmacopeia that included Balm of Gilead Bud. Taking their place were reams of biochemical, physiologic and pathologic knowledge *and* potent chemotherapeutic

agents. The emphasis on "the healer" in the old legend became paramount. Patients no longer expected sympathy and hand holding for their "double-pneumonia," but cures, and anticipated receiving a "shot of penicillin" or one of the miracle drugs that appeared in rapid succession.

Not only medicine changed, but all of society. The rural areas were slowly and inexorably abandoned. Cities grew larger and were surrounded by burgeoning suburbs. Family life changed as societal mobility increased. Gone were "grandpop" and "grandmom" sitting in the rocking chair in the corner while two or three or more generations lived shoulder to shoulder. The economy, government, religion and virtually every other institution underwent revolutionary change.

Yet legends die hard, and some never seem to die at all. Everyone remembered the kindly, old, home-visiting general practitioner. Few remembered his diagnostic and therapeutic impotence. Unfavorable comparison was drawn between the legend and the new crop of young men and women with syringe and prescription pad in hand who labored solely in a sparkling office and disdained home visits. Patients thought and felt they were being treated as objects or diseases or parts of the body in an assembly line medical production plant.

Thus derived the criticism of modern medicine as dehumanizing. It was too cerebral an activity, too intellectual. Where was the warmth of "old Mr. Jones' ulcer" instead of "that fascinating gastric ulcer" which just happened to reside in Mr. Jones' body? Somehow people seemed to be left out of medicine. It was now a study of processes, organs, tissues, cells, molecules and electrons. But not of people.

Unfortunately, this phenomenon has crept into medical education, reasoning and problem solving. Students of medicine were confronted by vast amounts of facts which had to be grasped, retained and regurgitated. Educators, once the kindly old physicians themselves, became bright-eyed and bushy-tailed young men and women who were pursuing truth as they also taught medicine. Medical schools became havens for some of the most competent bioscientists ever to have lived. Curricula quickly reflected these trends and became compartmentalized into rigid segments which treated that portion of medical knowledge exhaustively and in isolation from other portions. One didn't learn medicine; one learned biochemistry, pathology, obstetrics, psychiatry and all the other components.

Practice also reflected the change. General practioners became the minority; specialty practice became the mode. Further and further fragmentation occurred until finally one could specialize in the diagnosis and treatment of the retina!

Students were caught up in these trends and learned that it took extensive knowledge and skill to be a generalist—there simply was too much to know and apply. Why not wrap your intellectual arms completely around an area you could master, for example, the retina or the breast or the rectum! In the process some students lost sight of people for their parts. Such students became practitioners with attitudes and practices reflecting this distorted vision. They began to see "backs" and "hearts" and "ulcers" and "colds" streaming into their offices, rather than people. Some patients contributed by demanding narrow care confined to their ailment. After all, they were "busy" and needed to be mended to carry on their "busyness." So give them the pills and the shots, and they'll come back with the next problem. Never mind the complete examination—don't even bother to disrobe them.

From all of these trends have come modern medical practice and the focus that Percy brought to his studies. He had learned ideas, concepts, facts and tests and had ignored people. It really was easy to do, given our current society and medical educational approaches. He, and others, never "really thought about that" or "got the point." This book is an attempt to get the students to think about medicine as the practice of a discipline involving people and their problems. It does not ignore the importance of factual knowledge or skill but places them into a perspective that involves people.

We are not puzzle solvers for the sake of intellectual satisfaction. Nor are we computers with input-output data mechanically responding with the dispensation of healing. We are physicians whose function it is to help people solve problems arising in their bodies and minds. We cannot do so without knowledge, but that knowledge is a tool to accomplish a larger purpose; it is not an end unto itself. There is ample room in society and in medicine for theoreticians. We could not survive without them. But clinical practice is not theoretical. That does not mean it is nonintellectual or disdainful of theory. It simply means that intellect and theory must be brought to bear upon individual personal health problems. One aim of this book is to encourage you to always use your intellect and your knowledge in your practice; to make the scientific method a part of your everyday behavior rather than an activity confined to dark chambers and subhuman animals in a research institution. Physicians are selected, intelligent individuals capable of the highest degree of intellectual activity. This book is a plea for you to learn to use this talent maximally and with compassion and sensitivity.

What does a doctor actually do? By my definition he solves problems that people have as a result of some malfunction of their body. In this concept all of a physician's behavior is directed towards this goal, no matter how simple the activity, how mundane the task or how routine the procedure. If he is "treating" patients, he's solving problems. To do so requires certain components dealt with in detail in subsequent chapters of this book. An outline of the process and its attendant skills and attitudes is given in Chapter 2.

There are certain aspects of medicine deserving of fuller treatment in the context of clinical problem solving: (1) the need to reach decisions, often with little patient-contact time; (2) dependence on others to provide data; (3) the need for effective communication; and (4) preservation of the understanding of the patient.

One skill the physician must acquire is the ability to extract data, see the problem(s) and offer recommendations in a relatively short period of time. In short, he must develop efficiency. Conservation of time means he can insure his economic stability, he can avoid waste of the patient's time and he can offer his services to the many who require them. He must be efficient without sacrifice of accuracy or humanity. The only way to achieve this is by constant practice and a conscious effort at improvement. The beginning student is naturally slow and cumbersome as he acquires skills and knowledge. He finds that he speeds up to the degree that he is sure of his skills and to the extent of retained knowledge as he passes through the various stages of medical education and practice. Thus the emphasis on competence of skills and recall and use of knowledge. Students (and educators) should worry less about scores or grades on exams and view them more as diagnostic indicators of areas of deficit in the storage, retention or retrievability of knowledge.

As he acquires efficiency, effort is required to remain sensitive to the person from whom he is extracting data. Efficiency should not mean a cold, mechanical approach as a mental checklist of tasks is automatically performed. Rather, the physician becomes efficient by committing the skills to his behavior pattern so that they are automatic as his attention is devoted to the person. Throughout this book I will refer figuratively to a physician's or student's "antennae." The analogy with the insect or crustacean organ is a good one, since these creatures use them to "sense" their environment. In the same way, your figurative antennae should be tuned to the people you treat, your patients. Sensitivity to mood, affect, expression, so-called "body language," fear, anxiety, apprehension and the other countless forms of humanness evident in your patient will result in more effective data collection, better judgmental analysis of values of symptoms, and sounder practical therapeutic recommendations. In addition, you will enjoy greater patient confidence, since their antennae will detect your interest directed to them as persons.

Simple acts, such as looking directly at your patients, listening to them rather than speaking, seeking their reaction prior to painful probing, and the like, will reinforce in patients' minds your sincere concern and regard for them as individuals. In my experience the doctor-patient relationship that is founded on mature respect is the most effective. The doctor demonstrates his respect by such actions as the ones above because he does respect the patient. Most patients detect this respect. They also are quick to recognize aloofness, diffidence, indifference and all other manifestations of an impersonal relationship. Nor does the doctor have to verbalize these attitudes; simple body language suffices. The impatient tapping of a pencil while the patient speaks, the not too furtive glances at the wristwatch, the hurried, indifferent examination oblivious to the discomfort it produces, the patronizing gesture, the unanswered telephone call, the gazing into the middle distance because the physician's thoughts are elsewhere, all speak eloquently of the physician's attitude. Verbalizations such as, "I can only spend 5 minutes today; now what's your problem?" are obvious, but more subtle expressions also get across the sentiment that initiated them.

Sensitivity does not mean the substitution of friendliness for objectivity, knowledge or skill. It simply implies that the latter will be carried out with concerned competency. Nothing is less appropriate than the feeling of some physicians that expression of mature respect towards a patient demeans the professional attitude. There is nothing intrinsic to medicine that insists that the doctor be a cold, aloof authoritarian. It is true that in some situations for all patients, and most of the time in some patients, the physician's effectiveness is based upon command and decisiveness. But these are exceptional circumstances; they are utilized more as tools of the professional to accomplish some objective and not as a device to diminish the patient's importance in the relationship.

Efficiency, therefore, implies a competency expressed in brevity with little lost motion and no loss in sensitivity and compassion.

A second characteristic of clinical encounters is the utter dependence upon the patient or a relative or other interested nonprofessional party to implement the physician's recommendations. In many diagnostic or treatment plans the physician will prescribe a course of action and assess future events as if that course of action were carried out scrupulously. It is naive of a professional to expect that following a brief encounter an untrained nonprofessional will follow a prescribed set of activities with perfection. Therefore, he must take steps to insure that this will occur. A great deal of the success of this effort stems from effective communication, which will be dealt with subsequently and more fully. Another factor in success is the effective utilization of paraprofessionals to complement and extend the instructions, i.e., to be a communicator. An office nurse, a trained receptionist, a physician's assistant or whomever the doctor designates and trains can provide a link to the patient that amplifies and augments the prescribed actions desired. More important than who does it is the basic understanding of the doctor that his professional advice needs interpretation to the patient. On many items he can provide the interpretation to the patient. One useful device is to write out or have prepared all instructions. There are many others. Use of such devices indicates that the doctor understands the problem of unfamiliar actions by an untrained person.

In the evaluation of the effects of a treatment plan the physician must remain a friendly skeptic. He must insure that what he prescribed was done, *before* he ascribes success or failure to the prescription (and to his problem-solving approach).

In actions requiring long-term performance he must often enlist the aid of a highly skilled technician who can teach the behavior and monitor it, even in the home, if necessary. There are many old hoary medical jokes that poke fun at long-term misapplication of physicians' instructions. Funny in the telling and hearing, they are far from humorous in a real patient.

A third, and perhaps the most critical, factor is effective communication. Few of us can accept the technical jargon associated with many specialized activities, such as space technology, government, architecture or even automobile mechanics, without lay interpretation. Little wonder that our highly technical discipline, medicine, also requires interpretation to the laity. Nowhere in medicine is this more evident than in the communication between doctor and patient. Accustomed to reading, thinking and expressing technical language, the physician must abruptly switch to ordinary English to be understood by his patients. "Ambulate" must become "walk," "respiratory" must become "chest" or "lungs," "otitis media" must become "ear infection," and so on. Even more critical than disease designation is the ultimate instruction to the patient. A pertinent study points this out, and some of the conclusions are worthy of highlight here.* The study evaluated the results of an encounter for children with otitis media. Less than half of the parents knew anything about the diagnosis, 68% did *not* know which antibiotic was administered, and 93% did not know what the decongestant was. A significant number did not know the functions of the various medications. The study further described the difficulties patients encountered in obtaining prescriptions, the marked variability in the dose administered, and the length of time that therapy was continued. If a simple acute illness, otitis media, results in such massive misinformation or lack of information, and in such variable practical pharmacology, what then of complex illnesses with long-term duration and multiple modalities of therapy?

The physician must insure that his patients understand the nature of their illness in at least general terms. This knowledge is often the sole motivating influence in carrying out therapy. Further, the physician must insure that his patients understand the therapy he prescribes, its rationale, the necessity to report difficulties or adverse effects and, finally, the ability to implement it. All of this depends upon effective communication. It is insufficient to reach a diagnosis, mumble its Latin name and hand the patient three or four prescriptions and turn to the next problem. It is a common occurrence that following such an encounter the patient either fails to fill the prescriptions or only partially fills them and subsequently administers them in a haphazard, incomplete fashion. All the intellectual

---

* Mattar, ME, et al: Inadequacies in the pharmacologic management of ambulatory children. *J. Pediatrics* 87:137–141, 1975.

"beauty" of the physician's competence is wasted in his failure to insure adequate compliance.

How can we communicate effectively? First, recognize the "jargon gap" between you and your patient. Second, take the time yourself or delegate the task to a reliably trained assistant. Third, the explanation must be in ordinary English, clearly and unequivocally phrased. "He has an infection caused by germs in the inside part of his right ear" is specific, is in lay terms, and helps the patient to understand the etiology, location and nature of the problem. Followed with, "It won't go away by itself. It can get worse, and the pus inside can burst the eardrum. This could hurt his hearing. He must be given this medicine (indicate name) which will kill the germs. It doesn't kill all of them right away, so it has to be taken for 1 week, every day. If it isn't, the germs can grow again, and the pain and fever will come back", and so on. If the disease demands equivocation, make this clear. "His sore throat may be due to germs which we call strep and which penicillin will kill. But it is possible that tinier germs, viruses, can be causing it, in which case the penicillin won't help. So I'm taking a swab of the pus in his throat, and the lab will tell me if strep germs are there and if he needs penicillin." Clear, concise, straightforward language. "Germs" is understood by most people; "bacteria" is not, and "streptococci" is understood by even fewer people.

Fourth, have the patient repeat your explanation. This simple exercise can be very humbling and will point up those instances when you've really failed to get your message across.

Fifth, use written material whenever practical and feasible. For repetitively encountered problems a well prepared, brief printed message can reinforce your verbal account. For individual situations you can *print* or legibly write out your instructions.

Sixth, establish some system of checking. The most frequent device is to have one of the office personnel talk to the patients on the telephone during the course of therapy. Alternatively, if you are certain the information was initially understood, you can instruct the patient to call if certain preselected events transpire.

The brevity and efficiency of most patient encounters may result in loss of the patient's individuality. This must be avoided. Just as you would not wish to be considered just another doctor, so the patient does not wish the anonymity of being "an ulcer" or "the 10-o'clock appointment" or whatever impersonalization comes to mind. Your patients are people with names, personalities, troubles and egos. They should be treated as unique individuals, not just another unit of your medical assembly line. Develop a personal style, as detailed previously. You are basically interested in and concerned for your patients as people. Let it show. Let them know that you recognize them as individuals. Never permit their disease or finding to replace their personal identity. I've heard one physician call his colleague into an examining room with the exclamation, "Hey, Joe, come and feel this spleen. It's huge!" Apart from the privacy that was invaded by the remark, it is a tasteless expression that reduced the person to an interesting organ to be exhibited. There is so much opportunity for this to happen in medical practice that the physician must be constantly on guard to discipline himself and those around him to resist the many temptations.

For a few patients in most practices something more than an ambulatory encounter will be needed; hospitalization will result. This practice should encompass all of the principles discussed previously, and they will not be repeated here. Only those characteristics unique to hospital practice will be explored.

The first decision faced by the physician is when to refer the patient to the hospital. In a few situations it takes little thought. Severe illness necessitating 24-hour professional care, certain instances of trauma, many surgical procedures, pregnancy and certain diagnostic procedures virtually mandate admission to hospital. In many instances the decision is not that simple. It is difficult to draw strict guidelines. Many factors enter such a decision: the nature of the disease, the severity and prognosis, the nature of the patient and his ability to be cared for at home, and the nature of the contemplated diagnosis and treatment. The physician makes an individual assessment of all of these factors. The trend today is to second-guess the physician in order to decrease the spiraling cost of inpatient care. Peer review of each hospital admission is being implemented to gauge the necessity for and the duration of hospitalization. Some rigid guidelines are being drawn up, and some measures to allow flexibility are being provided. It is difficult to project the final outcome of this development.

Assuming that the decision has been made to admit a patient to the hospital, what then? First, the physician must recognize what this dislocation does to the individual. Reactions vary from fear of impending death to joy at the release from daily responsibility. These reactions can influence the course of the patient, the response to therapy, and the degree of cooperation and must be assessed.

Second, the purposes of hospitalization must be clearly formulated and some plan developed to implement these goals. The nature of the inpatient encounter presupposes a more lengthy opportunity for evaluation. In contrast to the office visit, data can be more fully obtained and with somewhat greater leisure. This is especially true when physicians are available on a full-time basis at the hospital (e.g., residents or hired staff). The patient in the hospital offers multiple opportunities for questioning and reexamination. Observations of a longitudinal nature, such as blood pressure, urine output, glucosuria and seizure activity can be made by trained professionals. Response to therapy can be gauged accurately over time, from minute to minute or at longer intervals. Therapy can be carried out with reasonable assurance of precision and timing. All of these advantages should be accomplished under the aegis of a comprehensive, well-thought-out plan.

Third, hospitalization affords the opportunity for ease in consultation. Rather than the patient having to seek out a variety of physicians and professionals at their offices or institutional sites, these individuals can focus on the patient. This presents an opportunity for an orchestrated diagnostic analysis or therapeutic plan.

Fourth, care must be taken to avoid the inefficiency of hospitalization. A poorly formulated plan or lapses in implementation can result in prolonged stay. This exacerbates the patient's separation from routine life, increases the costs and impairs utility of the hospital bed.

For most physicians, hospital practice constitutes only a small portion of their total effort. For some it is a constant part of their practice, and for a few their practices are limited to hospital-based activities. For the vast majority of patients, hospitalization represents but a brief interlude in any given illness. Regardless of the physician's orientation to the hospital environment, he should always be mindful of the patient's attitude and perception. Hospital stays should not be prolonged and should not be utilized if outpatient diagnosis or care can be maintained.

The hospital stay of a patient also offers an unusual opportunity to educate or reeducate the patient. Instructions can be explained or reinforced. Observation of patient performance in the taking or administering of drugs (e.g., insulin injection) or in the performance of manipulative activities (e.g., urine testing for glucose, pulmonary toilet, exercises) can be easily accomplished and serve as a check on home performance. Whenever possible, hospitalization should be utilized in this way. It may be the only method of control in an otherwise-underserved patient activity.

In this chapter we have attempted to give an historic outlook to medical practices and both the professional and lay perceptions of the doctor and his functions. In addition, an outline of why and how the doctor functions in his environment has been sketched. The remainder of the book will concentrate upon those specific activities involved in the major function of a physician, problem solving. It should not be lost on the reader that the topics covered in this initial chapter *will* often determine if problem solving is a realistic activity of benefit to the patient, rather than an intellectual exercise.

Chapter 2

Clinical Problem Solving— What Is It?

Unfortunately, medicine is subject to the plight of all human disciplines; it becomes mired in its own jargon and cliches. One of these is encountered in the phrase "clinical problem solving." This shorthand expression has been used so frequently in recent years that, to some, it has lost its meaning. I will use this phrase throughout this book, since a more convenient, concise expression for the process to be discussed has not suggested itself.

DATA

For convenience I have depicted the clinical problem-solving process as a directional flow from data to action (see Fig. 2.1). In greatly simplified fashion this flow diagram indicates that the clinician collects data, forms explanations for their presence, tests his formulations and decides upon some course of action. Shown as clearly separate stages in the diagram, the process actually blends in practice. Hypotheses are formed as data are collected, testing may occur before final hypothesis formulation, and even clinical action is taken before solution of the "problem," in some instances. To better understand the process, I have chosen to dissect it into its components, artificially isolating the four major segments.

The practice of medicine is complex and embodies many skills—some scientific and technical, others more of "art" or "style." The central issue confronting most physicians in their daily encounters with patients is the resolution of some "problem" that the patient presents in the form of a series of statements or symptoms. Thus the process we are exploring usually begins with an encounter initiated because an individual "feels" unwell.

It is critical to explore this starting point with all of its ramifications. No attempt to "solve" patients' "problems" can begin without an appreciation of the patients' perceptions and just what these "data" are. Data are detailed in Chapter 3.

Having obtained a "history" from the patient, the physician completes his initial process by examining the patient. Physical examination and diagnosis are also discussed in Chapter 3.

HYPOTHESES

Having received all of the initial data, the physician begins the formal process known as "problem solving," or so it seems. Actually he has begun with his first contact with the patient. This is an extremely important point often lost on the initiate. He observes a good diagnostician and believes the process begins with the discussion of the differential diagnosis when, in fact, it, has already proceeded through many steps prior to the formulation of stated diagnoses. An example might help to place this point in its proper perspective.

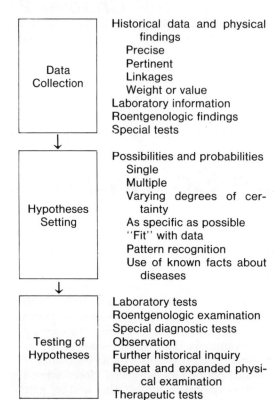

| Data Collection | Historical data and physical findings
Precise
Pertinent
Linkages
Weight or value
Laboratory information
Roentgenologic findings
Special tests |

| Hypotheses Setting | Possibilities and probabilities
Single
Multiple
Varying degrees of certainty
As specific as possible
"Fit" with data
Pattern recognition
Use of known facts about diseases |

| Testing of Hypotheses | Laboratory tests
Roentgenologic examination
Special diagnostic tests
Observation
Further historical inquiry
Repeat and expanded physical examination
Therapeutic tests |

| Action or Inaction | Specific to hypotheses
To return patient to homeostatic balance |

Figure 2.1. Components of the problem-solving process.

A 6-week-old male infant presented with intractable vomiting of 4-weeks' duration. Initially a minor problem, the vomiting has become severe, with complete emptying of the stomach contents after each feeding. There has been associated weight loss and increasing lethargy in the past 2 weeks.

To the inexperienced a discussion of this problem might seem to begin following examination and without laboratory data. The student is usually exposed to the diagnostician at this point and perceives the subsequent steps in the "differential diagnosis" of vomiting in early infancy. In fact, the process began with the first phone call the physician received from the parents. The process of establishing hypotheses was initiated even as the mother related the events of the past 4 weeks. Had the physician been thinking aloud, we might have heard the following or a close facsimile:

"There's nothing in the prenatal or birth history to suggest onset of a process that was acquired *in utero* or at delivery. Could he have been infected in the nursery? He might be septic. On the other hand, his illness has been prolonged and, although serious, does not seem to be fulminant enough for most neonatal bacterial infections. I must look for possible signs of intrauterine viral disease that may be manifesting itself this late. He is a male, and I don't recall anything about his genitalia to suggest adrenal problems. Could he be obstructed? She's telling me his vomiting is very forceful and has soiled his room because of its expulsive force. On the other hand, he probably has simple gastroenteritis, but I'd better check him, since his symptoms are so severe and he's just a young infant."

What has occurred is a constant testing of the data *as it is collected.* These early thoughts may be totally afield or right to the mark. It doesn't matter at this point. What is critical is that the data are being "weighed." Data are being sifted according to the knowledge, experience and wisdom of the sifter. To a beginning student, age and sex and symptoms may carry equal significance or may seem to be totally unrelated. It's as if a civilian was asked to look over a field of sophisticated military hardware. An intelligent observer might note all of the equipment and pieces of equipment lying about and could faithfully describe them in writing, but one piece has the same significance as another. If a military equipment expert surveys the same scene, he will rapidly categorize the equipment by several different criteria. The significant difference between these observers is *not* intelligence or power of observation, but specific knowledge of a systematized scheme for organizing information. Similarly, "experience" or "wisdom" in medicine is a deft combination of intelligence plus knowledge of the systems of medicine which help us to organize information regarding health and disease. To use our example and oversimplify, a student perceives a 6-week-old male infant and vomiting as separate entities, whereas the clinician recognizes that in his particular medical universe there are several *linkages* to these seemingly isolated bits of data. He knows that certain disease processes (infections, endocrinopathies, intestinal obstruction and others) occur among many 6-week-old male infants. He also knows that certain other diseases either do *not* occur in this population or occur with such rarity that they need not be considered at first blush. Simply stated, he "knows" the current systematization of the medical world we live in. Further, he can apply the data in the present case to the system in general, and vice versa.

This long discussion serves to illustrate the first major point in understanding what is meant by "problem solving"; "data" (symptoms, signs, laboratory analyses, etc.) are not random, isolated bits of information but are expressions of natural phenomena. The point of this concept is that we become good "problem solvers" (1) to the extent that the natural order is understood by medicine as a whole and (2) to the degree to which the individual perceives what is understood about nature.

Such concepts are obvious but escape many students and residents who are in pursuit of clinical competence. Rather than trying to understand pathophysiology and generalize from it and specify from the generalization, the student may seek simply to "remember" associations, lists of diseases, or symptom correlations. The student then is puzzled when a more experienced observer can think through a problem following natural pathophysiologic associations. The clinician appreciates the natural world about him and how disease causes deviations from health. He views the data bits as clues or cues to the underlying pathophysiology. To return to our example, the clinician knows that infants are subject to certain environmental influences at different ages. He knows that these influences produce a limited number of bodily responses. He knows that the responses produce a limited number of perceivable and observable symptoms and signs. The degree to which he knows these facts is the degree to which he is a "good" diagnostician.

The understanding that medicine as a scientific discipline has achieved in describing the limits referred to above will dictate to a great extent just how "good" any diagnostician can be. If a disease process is poorly understood, and if its effects on the body are still unpredictable and diverse, we refer to its manifestations as "protean" or to the disease as a "great imitator," or we employ some other conceit which really says we don't completely know what's going on!

A good example in today's practice is systemic lupus erythematosus. We do not know its etiology and are still exploring the many facets of its manifestations. As a result, it is a disease which frequently escapes detection early in its course and which may defy resolution even by the most astute observers. If one looks into an older textbook of medicine, one can find that acute streptococcal pharyngitis, syphilis and tuberculosis once were in an almost identical position as lupus is today. When the causes of these diseases were unknown and the pathophysiology uncertain, doctors were befuddled by the signs and symptoms, and the processes resulted in "protean" manifestations. As we learned what caused them and the effects of the particular infectious agent became clear, these diseases moved closer to predictable entities which could be recognized more easily than previously.

Whether one accepts that the diagnostic process begins upon first contact or not, it is obvious that at some point hypotheses are developed which best "fit" the available data. Such hypotheses function as testable explanations of the process(es) occurring in the patient. As indicated above, early hypotheses are discarded or retained based upon the accumulation of information. During the course of thinking through a specific problem there occurs a time or times when the data are sufficiently abundant to allow formation of an explanation. This is usually in the form of a statement of probability. The data may be so all-encompassing as to lead to a single, highly probable or almost certain hypothesis; or many explanations may occur to the diagnostician of varying probability; or anything in between. Literally, the data plus the knowledge of the observer dictate the extent, variety and exactness of hypothesis formation.

The formulation of an hypothesis and the accuracy in determining how many need to be formed with what degree of probability constitutes a central skill in problem solving.

An anecdote or two may help to emphasize this point.

During the writing of this book our family cat, Confetti, provided an example of random data collection and total inability to form an hypothesis. This is roughly comparable to the beginnings of the process in humans. Confetti is, like most cats, an inquisitive observer of her environment. She discovered mirrors at an early age and, regardless of the environment or the height or massiveness of the mirror, seeks out any reflective surface as a primary objective wherever she happens to be. Her skill at finding mirrors is unparalleled. It requires curiosity, agility, good eyesight, and recognition of a reflecting surface (i.e., good data collection associated with the necessary physical abilities to obtain the data). Having done all of this repeatedly in diverse environments, she then proceeds to scratch repeatedly on the surface of the mirror, presumably in an attempt to get at the cat she sees there who makes identical movements towards her. She cannot form an hypothesis which tested once (or twice or even three times) could be verified or denied. She probably will go on attempting to communicate physically with her mirror image as long as her faculties hold out.

Confetti illustrates at once the plight of many beginners in clinical medicine and a few clinicians. She is "stuck" despite her superior data collection because she cannot form an hypothesis or, rather, because she forms a faulty one and persists in its testing despite the seemingly obvious answer she gets. How like the student who having learned interviewing and physical examination techniques applies these to a patient who is ill, collects his data and then is "stuck," or the physician who insists that the diagnosis he has "established" is the correct one despite the repeated negative results of testing. The difference between these individuals and Confetti is that they need not look forward to a lifetime of similar pursuit, while she does!

Establishing hypothesis is as much an art as it is a science. But the artfulness need not place a mystique upon the process. The elements of the art are within almost every student of medicine and, further, can be polished and applied without resort to magic or invocation of godlike powers.

This innate ability *can* be developed and polished. The only certain way to accomplish increasing skill is by some form of experience. You must practice this skill repeatedly and in a critical fashion. You must profit by both your faculty contacts and by your patient encounters. You must think. One cannot learn this skill or develop it in clinical medicine by "osmosis" alone. You must force yourself or be forced to use it constantly. Even with simple, obvious problems one must, in the beginning, analyze why he has reached his conclusion. With more complicated clinical problems the necessity for such exercise becomes more obvious and thus more frequently achieved, but not always, since it is too easy to become slothful.

In a protected environment (such as medical school or a residency program) it is relatively easy to allow the thinking of those about you to replace all or part of your own. You must avoid this easily adapted behavior. There are several ways to do this. First, upon collecting your own data, form an opinion. Do not rush to the nearest intern, resident or faculty member to peek at their conceptualization. Second, having formulated your opinion, be absolutely critical in analyzing it in contrast to those about you. Third, follow your patient's course and evaluation of the problem in order ultimately to measure your thinking against actual clinical events. Fourth, as you progress in your responsibility, avoid the pitfalls of diagnostic manual medicine. That is, do not substitute a readily available list in some shorthand textbook for your own analysis. The busy intern and resident find time to be so consumed with doing things that they often fail to think. Many such individuals come to rely on some shorthand method which has the long-term effect of delaying and even aborting the thinking process.

Fifth, ask each clinician you come into contact with why he reached the conclusions he did about a particular case. Find out what the elements of his hypothesis setting were. Why did he reject what seemed to be a reasonable alternative? Why did he set three (or X) possibilities? Why did he choose to test Hypotheses 1 and 2 first and hold 3 in reserve? And so on. It is not sufficient for clinicians simply to expose the ultimate result of their thinking. If they are to participate in your education, it is important that the answers to questions of the above type be provided to you. Your job is to insist upon it, courteously and politely and with due regard to the setting and timing of the discussion, but to insist upon it, nonetheless. You can gain valuable insight into the way clinicians solve problems by such interactions, the *how* and *why* of the solution. This complements the more-usually-available *what*.

Let us return to our clinical example to see if these principles can be applied to a specific instance. The clinician who is confronted with the 6-week-old male who is vomiting will most likely establish the following hypotheses: (1) obstructive intestinal process, (2) systemic infection, (3) endocrinopathy and (4) gastroenteritis.

Without saying so, he will have rejected, outright, hematologic, malignant, traumatic, topic and other etiologic categories and will have ranked metabolic and noninfectious inflammatory causes to a secondary, more remote ranking. Why? And how?

First, he will appreciate that in the universe of the 6-week-old, certain disease processes are prevalent and can result in vomiting. Second, he knows that the *pattern* of illness, i.e., the linkage and sequence of the symptoms observed, are consistent with known diseases because of their high probability (more of this later).

Thus, during the extension of data collection—additional history and physical examination—he will first explore these known conditions. He is seeking a summation of clues which by their pattern will suggest confirmatory tests. In this example he will find them. In others he will not, and we will subsequently explore such an instance.

As he obtains the history he will ask about the mother's health during pregnancy (the possibility of intrauterine infection) and the infant's neonatal period (looking for evidence of disordered feeding, elimination or behavior, for fever and/or localized signs of infection), he will carefully document the already volunteered symptoms (to establish their exact character and relationships with other events to see if a pattern is evident), and he will then assess, at an age-appropriate level, the presence or absence of other symptoms (review of systems).

Satisfying himself that the dimensions of the clinical difficulty have been adequately explored at this stage, he will proceed to examine the infant. Despite the fact that a "complete" physical examination occurs, he will focus most intently upon those areas of the body which are likely to express underlying infections, structural or endocrinologic pathophysiologic changes.

In the example given, the physician noted (1) a relatively unresponsive infant when undisturbed; (2) sudden and generalized irritability upon examination, particularly when the abdomen was palpated; (3) dry skin which was devoid of the usual elasticity; (4) dry mucous membranes; (5) no tears; (6) no observable urination during examination; (7) no obvious infectious focus (mucous membranes, umbilicus, penis, lungs); (8) no pigmentary changes in the penis or scrotum; (9) a flat abdomen which was distended in the epigastrium following glucose water feeding; and (10) the presence of an ill-defined mass deep in the epigastrium in the midline; bowel sounds and percussion of the abdomen were normal.

These findings were elicited partially as a result of a careful total examination and partially because they were being specifically sought. The reasoning underlying the search was as follows:

"Regardless of the cause, certain imbalance in homeostasis can be expected by such protracted vomiting. Therefore, I must look for signs of fluid loss and electrolyte imbalance (thus the focus upon the state of hydration). The history suggests several prominent possibilities. First, *systemic severe infection.* Therefore, I must explore the possibility of meningitis, otitis media, pneumonia and urinary tract infection at a minimum. Second, *structural abnormality.* It is possible that obstruction of the intestinal tract is present; therefore, I must carefully examine the abdomen for signs of distension, for physiologic abnormalities and for disturbed structure (e.g., masses or distended loops of bowel). And third, *endocrinopathy.* Variants of adrenal hyperplasia are most likely here. Is there evidence for excess androgen production from the adrenal? (Hence the scrutiny of the scrotum and penis for signs of disproportionate maturity.)"

It is important to note the directed approach of this physician. He is *constantly thinking through his patient's problem*, and his data collection technique and intensity are *directed* and not random. Having established hypotheses with high probability, he *first* tests them. At the same time he does not ignore the possibility that he is wrong and a different cause is responsible. He guards against this by being reasonably complete, although not necessarily exhaustibly so. This is a sound approach to clinical problem solving but not the only one. Let us examine some alternatives at this point.

The physician could have chosen to gather a "complete" history and do a "complete" physical examination without regard to hypotheses. Although many medical educators (including me) have preached the virtues of this approach and countless thousands of students have been taught to practice it, it is not the *usual* way problems are attacked. But it is an alternative, and for some clinical situations is the only, and the correct, choice. This is especially true for those problems which do not readily suggest hypothesis (e.g., the manifestations cannot easily be linked, *or* they are so few and nonspecific as to be possibly due to a myriad of causes, *or* they are unfamiliar to the physician). In these instances a thorough approach is critical, since evidence of the pathophysiologic processes may be found in virtually any organ, tissue or system. Only completeness will insure that the physician has the best data to utilize.

An extension of this approach is the consideration of *all* reasonable hypotheses. This method is the common *differential diagnostic approach.* In our example, all reasonable causes of vomiting in infancy would be listed. The usual approach is to rely on some all-inclusive system of disease. Such systems include anatomic, etiologic or physiologic organization of knowledge (Tables 2.1 to 2.3). Hence one might consider as etiologic categories infections, metabolic, structural, congenital, traumatic, malignant, immunologic and so on until all possible known categories are included. Then an additional category is added, such as "idiopathic" or "miscellaneous," to include those possibilities that do

Table 2.1
Etiologic Classification of Diseases

Allergic
Congenital
Endocrinologic
Genetic
Hematologic
Idiopathic
Immunologic
Infectious
Iatrogenic
Malignant
Metabolic
Miscellaneous
Nutritional
Psychosocial
Toxic
Traumatic

Table 2.2
Anatomic Classification of Diseases

Cardiovascular system
Dental
Endocrinologic organs
Gastrointestinal tract
Genitourinary system
Hematopoietic system
Immunologic system
Multisystem disorders
Muscular system
Nervous system
Respiratory tract and mediastinum
Reticuloendothelial system
Skeletal system
Skin and appendages
Special sensory organs

Table 2.3
Pathophysiologic Classification of Diseases

Aging processes
Biochemical disorders
Circulatory disturbances
Degenerative disorders
Growth and development disorders
Idiopathic disorders
Inflammatory processes
Mechanical disruptions
Neoplasia
Nutritional disorders
Psychosocial disorders
Toxic disorders
Traumatic disorders

not neatly fit our attempts at etiologic pigeon-holing.

From among these categories are selected diseases or conditions which fit, or are fit, by the symptoms and signs of the patient. A "differential diagnosis" is generated. The degree of knowledge of the diagnostician coupled with his ability to assess probability will determine the length and the breadth of the list. One inherent problem with this approach is the tendency on the part of inexperienced diagnosticians to make the list too lengthy and too broad. I've termed this the "intern's syndrome," since its fruits can be encountered most frequently at the conclusion of a typical intern's "history and physical" (Fig. 2.2). In an attempt to be all-inclusive for his patient, his peers and his *mentors*, the intern tends to list all possible causes, no matter how remote. In some instances he doesn't even appreciate the remoteness of the possibilities listed, being unable to distinguish among "book" choices with which he has no familiarity or experience. The compulsive or insecure physician *at any level* may manifest the "intern's syndrome." It is fostered in some practices by a desire to not miss the correct diagnosis and in some medical educational institutions by the desire, conscious or unconscious, to display one's knowledge. In either instance it may not serve the patient very well. Since most clinical hypotheses are working explanations, they need to be tested. To make a long list of possibilities longer than it needs to be, results in the patient being possibly subjected to unnecessary, costly, uncomfortable or even dangerous diagnostic or therapeutic procedures.

The totality of the differential diagnostic approach can be modified if one assigns probabilities to the complete listing of possibilities. Then only those possibilities which are of high probability will be investigated initially. Sequential diagnosis then becomes possible, and the physician will go down his list in a logical fashion and, for most of his patients, will avoid unnecessary testing (Fig. 2.3). Of course, for a few patients the least probable will be the correct diagnosis. For these patients the efficacy of the sequential diagnostic system will be inefficient. In the balance, many more patients will benefit than will have delays in diagnosis.

I prefer the sequential approach and believe it is the most sophisticated and efficient way to practice medicine. Your patients will be the benefactors of a thoughtfully applied diagnostic approach based upon probability.

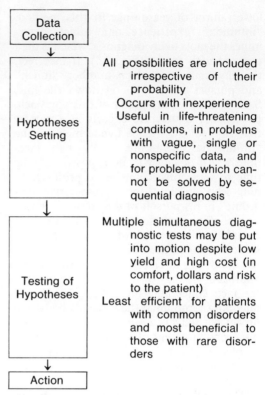

Figure 2.2. The intern's syndrome or differential diagnosis.

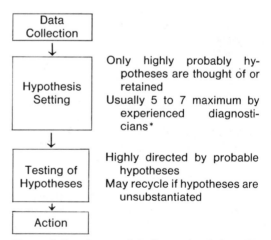

Figure 2.3. Sequential diagnosis. (*See Elstein, AS, Shulman, LS, and Sprafka, SA: *Medical Problem Solving: An Analysis of Clinical Reasoning.* Harvard University Press, Cambridge, MA, 1978.)

The final category of diagnostic approaches is mentioned for completeness but is to be condemned as poor practice and the lowest form of reasoning. In this method, "intuition," "experience" or a "hunch" determines the most likely diagnosis, which is then pursued with fervor (Fig. 2.4). If incorrect, the physician then selects another "hunch" and pursues it. And so on down the line. Some professors are guilty of this approach, particularly if they are experts in a narrow field of medicine. Hence I've termed this the "professorial syndrome," only half facetiously. All of you will be exposed at some time to some physician, be he professor or not, who employs the "professorial syndrome" in his pursuit of diagnoses. The caricature of the professor sweeping onto a ward, complete with a retinue of house officers and students ranked according to a strict hierarchy following in close pursuit, sums up this approach. He may or may not listen to all of the facts concerning the patient, he may or may not thump upon the patient's body, but he always delivers a monologue ending with his pronouncement of his diagnosis. Let me emphasize that this method is *not* limited to professors, and most professors do not employ it.

The essence of this approach is the assumption by the diagnostician that his expe-

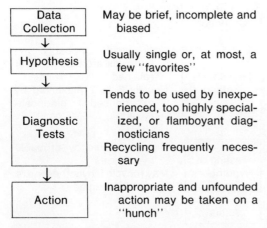

Data Collection	May be brief, incomplete and biased
Hypothesis	Usually single or, at most, a few "favorites"
Diagnostic Tests	Tends to be used by inexperienced, too highly specialized, or flamboyant diagnosticians Recycling frequently necessary
Action	Inappropriate and unfounded action may be taken on a "hunch"

Figure 2.4. The guess, intuitive or "professorial" approach to clinical problem solving. An expert diagnostician with rapid and correct analyses may appear to be using this technique, when, in fact, he is actually using sequential or differential diagnosis with rapid rejection of improbable hypotheses.

rience gives him some clairvoyant view of a patient's problem. This self-assurance leads to an intuitive approach in which an inner voice, recognizing some telltale correlation, speaks quickly and accurately. If the physician *is* both experienced *and* lucky, he may make some brilliant diagnosis, thereby cutting through all the red tape associated with a more thoughtful, if slower, approach. My suspicion is that the correct brilliant insights are remembered, whereas the incorrect conclusions and hunches tend to be submerged. One always remembers the luminous fiery comets that cross the sky and tends to disregard the billions of silent, unmoving stars that form the backdrop.

Some students succumb to the professorial syndrome early in their careers. They are usually intelligent, perceptive, intuitive individuals whose entire life has been focused on their quick-wittedness. They learn about clinical syndromes, they become very enthusiastic about their newfound knowledge, and soon everything becomes crystal-clear on first inspection. One such student became obsessed with systemic lupus erythematosus. Far in advance of his peers he learned of all the variations of this fascinating disease. Soon he invaded the wards, and *any* patient who had one of the many manifestations of this disease had lupus, unequivocally and without doubt! Despite many obvious errors, it took 2 years for him to settle into a more reasonable approach and for him not to see lupus on top of every hospital bed.

Less obvious examples of this kind of reasoning abound in medicine. Its very presence in many individuals, at one time or another, probably speaks to its origins. In a discipline in which uncertainty is encountered everywhere, how reassuring it is to seize upon some knowledge which can clearly be claimed as one's own. How convincing you can become if you know all there is to know about a limited subject. How easy then to shrug off uncertainty and "recognize" your disease or diseases amid the myriad of daily problems. Maturity in a physician can usually be measured by how he deals with uncertainty. A small digression into this phenomenon is warranted here.

That we do not know all there is to know

in medicine is a certainty that each of us needs to come face to face with at some point in our education. I once encountered a student who, upon contemplating the diagnostic method, decided that the process was silly and required too much unnecessary effort and was *uncertain*. His solution, which was obvious to him, was to select an entire battery of diagnostic tests, encompassing the majority of what was available in our routine laboratory, and apply it to *every* patient in the hospital. In this way, he said, we would almost never fail to detect a patient's problem, and what is more, we would save countless days in searching for the correct diagnosis. Apart from some practical consideration of multiphasic screening, further exploration of the student's thinking led to the conclusion that he was *frightened* about the uncertainties of medicine. He actually found terrifying the possibility that he would not reach a satisfactory conclusion in each and every patient with whose problems he dealt. Further, he did not wish to lose any time in reaching a conclusion, since this was inefficient and wasteful of his effort.

This encounter points up the dilemma that most of us face. We are not gods, we are not infallible, we are not even totally knowledgeable about our own discipline. We will be uncertain in specific instances, and we will encounter the frustration of not knowing in a good deal of our clinical work. The immature physician cannot believe this. He entered medicine with a rather naive view of the potency of the discipline, and he has not yet learned to cope with its darker sides. Most often he has not faced death in one of his patients; he has not stood beside a bed and watched some disease process whittling away at his patient's life with the realization that he has exhausted his and his colleagues' armaments; he has not encountered familiar signs and symptoms which should add up to a known process, but which do not; he has not tasted of the myriad moral and ethical dilemmas for which there are no textbook answers and for which he must rely upon his own resources and his patient's philosophy. He wants to be omnipotent, he wants to know everything, he wants to be able *always* to have some diagnostic or therapeutic maneu-

ver available, he wants to be able to do something. From this group of unrests he acts. And he does so with self-assurance. He is easy prey for the professorial syndrome.

The mature physician, on the other hand, meets all of the crises in medicine with equanimity and little or no frustration. He does not wish omniscience or omnipotence; he knows they are unattainable. Most of us are somewhere in between. We would like to be more than we can be but are realistic about our limitations. We would like never to experience frustration but know we will and do. But most importantly, we have learned to deal with uncertainty, with not knowing and with, sometimes, not doing anything. We have developed personal codes, beliefs and philosophies that permit us to deal with the moral and ethical dimensions of our practices. We know that we are human. We try to become good diagnosticians and think about the problems posed by our patients and attempt to solve them.

The diagnostic methods we've surveyed have some common features:

1. The best available data are obtained.
2. Each bit of data is as well defined as is possible.
3. Linkages between bits of data are recognized.
4. Hypotheses are formed to explain the appearance of the data in this specific patient.
5. Probabilities of hypotheses being correct are assigned.

Points 1, 2 and 3 will be fully discussed in Chapter 3. We've spent some time on Point 4, and it will be more fully discussed in Chapter 4.

Probability is axiomatic in the problem-solving process. The closest most of us get to probability theory is the knowledge that each flip of a coin has an even chance of coming up heads or tails. In clinical medicine we can usually do better than that. Probability in our discipline is related to *commonness*. This has been expressed concisely in the old saw that upon hearing hoofbeats in the night one thinks of horses, not zebras. Common processes in medicine occur commonly because they are common! Such an obvious statement may seem inappropriate and a put-down to readers. But it is not! Too frequently have we witnessed physicians searching for exotic diseases in their patients when even a cursory glance at their data suggests more usual problems. For every sore throat that is diphtheria, there are hundreds of thousands that are viral or streptococcal. For every instance of chest pain that signals hiatal hernia, there are thousands upon thousands that signal coronary insufficiency. And so on. Medical probability operates inexorably, since it is based upon a limited array of pathophysiologic responses to a limited number of noxious influences in the environment. When the medical coin is flipped, common things come up more frequently than do rare things.

Thus the diagnostician who is confronted with a set of symptoms, signs and laboratory data consistent with many possibilities is most often correct if he assumes that the commonest causes are operative—a simple concept, but one missed repeatedly in everyday practice activity. As physician-scientists we are fascinated by the exotic; as normal egotistic humans we are entranced with the opportunity to discover an odd disease.

The search for unique diseases is not as important universally as the commoner practice of "hedging your bets"—including just one or two diagnostic tests more than are necessary in order to catch that odd situation that may escape us. Such practice is costly to the patient, may be dangerous if the "just one or two tests" include those with risk, such as contrast studies, drug sensitivity tests or those employing nuclear medicine techniques. But the critical point is the unnecessary nature of their performance. Some examples may help to emphasize the daily employment of such thinking.

Children who experience febrile convulsions usually have no serious, underlying disease—"usually" in this case meaning almost always. Nevertheless, the "cautious" physician may hospitalize such a child and apart from the necessary history, physical, and possible examination of spinal fluid, will obtain a complete skull roentgenologic examination, a blood urea nitrogen, determination of calcium and phosphorus levels, a blood glucose level, urine examination for amino acids, and an electroencephalogram. If he is very insecure, he may even request neurologic consul-tation, and on occasion, this has resulted in the performance of computerized axial tomography or cerebral angiography, just to be sure (after all, if he called in a neurologist, the problem must be serious).

Let us examine the physician's choices in the light of current knowledge. Febrile seizures, without any unusual history or focal neurologic signs or unusual characteristics of the convulsion itself, occur almost exclusively in otherwise healthy children. On very, very rare occasions, a structural anomaly, a metabolic disease, a cerebral neoplasm (very rare in children) or renal disease may cause a child to have a febrile seizure as an initial manifestation. Less rare and of great personal risk to the patient is the occasional child who has purulent meningitis. These are facts clearly established in the medical body of knowledge, they have been taught for years and can be found in any standard textbook of pediatrics.

A thorough history and physical examination are mandatory, and many physicians would perform a lumbar puncture with a first febrile convulsion because of moderate probability of meningitis and because the risk of delayed diagnosis is considerable. Beyond that there is little rationale for further testing, if all historical and examination data are normal. Search for renal, metabolic and intracranial causes is fruitless in the overwhelming majority of instances. Certainly no one can justify the cost of CAT scans or the risk of cerebral angiography in such a setting, and few can offer sufficient justification for the other tests. But commonly in practice, such searches are made. Why? Because of substitution of a routine for thinking. Because of our insecurity. Because of an inflated sense of the risk of failing to do so. Because on rare occasions somebody does find something. The effect of one chance diagnosis upon local practice is astounding. Very quickly the news is spread, and almost as quickly the particular diagnostic test or procedure becomes the fad of that locale. The fact that a 1:10,000 chance of febrile seizure being due to a metabolic cause happens to operate in a particular physician-patient encounter does not justify metabolic screening in the 9,999 children in whom metabolic disease is not probable.

I do not wish to leave the impression that

one should always search for diseases of high probability in every situation. Often we are given clues to the presence of one of the processes with lesser probability. *In that patient who yields such clues the usually rare process becomes one of high probability.* An example is a child presenting with a febrile seizure, and on physical examination one finds hemangiomata on one side of the face in the distribution of the trigeminal nerve ophthalmic branch; then Sturge-Weber disease (encephalotrigeminal angiomatosis) becomes highly probable instead of a remote possibility on the tag end of everyone's differential diagnosis list of febrile seizures. A more subtle occurrence might be the history of pica (ingestion of dirt or other material) which may lead the clinician to vault lead poisoning from a low probability to a much higher one, necessitating screening tests even though the probability is not 100% in such instances.

In short, you must *think* about your patients' problems. Do not develop into a physician who surrounds himself with "routines" for certain conditions in his patient and who "always" gets this series of tests for this set of clinical clues. It is too easy to allow the routine to substitute for careful history taking and thorough examination.

An additional hazard awaits those who probe too widely, given their patient's symptoms and signs. They may find something! In fact, the something they find may be erroneous or a normal variant and not diagnostic of anything. But the physician is now forced to follow the false lead (he may not recognize it as false) and, at a minimum, repeat the test and, at a maximum, involve the patient in an expensive risky battery of unnecessary tests. The medical literature is rapidly expanding in the area of iatrogenic disease, a portion of which is due to overuse of diagnostic testing in situations which do not warrant it.

Knowledge of probability then is a critical factor in the problem-solving process. When one learns his facts he should also learn where that process fits into the entire fabric of medicine. You cannot treat renal tubular acidosis as equivalent to acute glomerulonephritis on the scale of probability. Again, one mustn't neglect those clues provided by one's patients which change the probability in the specific instance. But in the bulk of problems that confront one, commonness will usually rule.

TESTING CLINICAL HYPOTHESES

Hypotheses are established to be tested. If in our original problem, that of vomiting in the 6-week-old male, our hypotheses are (1) intestinal obstruction, probably pyloric stenosis, (2) severe systemic infection and (3) adrenal insufficiency due to adrenal hyperplasia, and we have assigned a high probability to pyloric stenosis (age, sex, course, physical findings), and a much lesser probability to sepsis and adrenal insufficiency, we can test the validity of the hypothesis. There are several possibilities: (1) we could obtain an examination of the upper gastrointestinal tract by contrast studies, (2) we could obtain consultation with a surgeon to both verify our findings or extend them and subsequently perform an exploratory laporatomy, or (3) we could sit the infant up, feed him a thickened formula and administer gastrointestinal relaxants. Each of these options has been and is being employed in identical circumstances to those of our patient. These alternatives serve to illustrate the major ways in which we test hypotheses.

First, and most commonly, we employ diagnostic laboratory techniques and tests to verify or deny our hypotheses. Perfect application of this principle would always result in a specific test or tests yielding a diagnostic result that was unequivocal. Few times in medicine do we reach this ideal. Most often we can confirm portions of the pathophysiologic processes consistent with our diagnosis. For example, we might detect casts, hematuria and albuminuria in a child with dark urine, edema and hypertension. With an extremely high degree of probability we have "diagnosed" acute glomerulonephritis (we really haven't, and unless we examine the glomeruli, we can't be absolutely sure that the process is glomerulonephritis). In fact, only with the application of special microscopic techniques can we reduce the uncertainty to a level of "almost certain" diagnosis. Of course, in most instances it is not essential to go this far. For most of our clinical problems, confirmatory evidence of the pathophysiologic alterations consistent with our main thesis is sufficient. We will explore the ramifications of diagnostic testing in Chapter 5.

A second alternative is to obtain an additional opinion(s). The time-honored method of consultation is employed. Under the conventional wisdom that two heads are better than one, we seek help in establishing a diagnosis from those who are better informed, more skillful or with more experience. This is another critical feature in the practice of medicine—the recognition of our limits. No one physician can be all things to all patients. We can become competent in our chosen subdiscipline within medicine and, by practicing thoughtfully, can serve most of our patients' needs. But we cannot serve all of them. We will establish our limits and learn which problems and which portions of certain problems require other physicians' advice. The inexperienced physician may think he feels the pyloric mass in our 6-week-old infant, but he may not be certain. If he has expert surgical consultation available, his hypotheses may be verified by the deft fingers of an experienced physician. There are so many examples of this phenomenon that I need not belabor it here.

The third alternative is the therapeutic trial. One can employ corrective therapy in situations where the hypothesis cannot be confirmed by laboratory techniques, *or* where the probability is very high that we are correct, *or* where the course of the disease is so fulminant that delay in therapy cannot be tolerated, *or* by any combination of these. Therapeutic trials can be diagnostic but may also be misleading. To cite my favorite example, a 6-year-old girl presented with fever (105 to 106° F), headache and a petechial rash confined to her ankles and wrists and the dorsum of her hands and feet. She lived in Colorado and had gone into the mountains with her family on many occasions. The presumptive hypothesis was that she had Rocky Mountain spotted fever. Diagnostic tests for this disease take some time to perform, and it was decided that the clinical evidence was so convincing that a therapeutic trial of tetracycline was warranted. She received this antibiotic for 1 week, during which she became afebrile, her headache subsided and her rash, which had extended somewhat at first,

faded into brown lesions (Fig. 2.5). Almost everyone was convinced that she had Rocky Mountain spotted fever and that the tetracycline had been curative. However, no organisms were isolated. She did not develop Proteus OX agglutinins, and no specific antibody was detected in her convalescent sera. This child had atypical measles which resulted from her prior inoculation of killed measles virus vaccine and which had altered her immunologic status and made her susceptible to wild virus exposure and a unique disease. And her case history made a convincing presentation for the efficacy of tetracycline in Rocky Mountain spotted fever. We were wrong! This young lady's problem illustrates clearly how the interpretation of therapeutic trials may be totally incorrect. There are countless examples in everyday practice.

Perhaps most common is the administration of antibiotics to an individual with a viral respiratory infection. Upon recovery we tend to associate the therapy with the cure and infer that the disease was bacterial. Many controlled trials have indicated the erroneous nature of this inference, and yet we still practice it—we choose not to *think*, but to *do*.

When correctly applied and interpreted, therapeutic trials can be doubly useful—they assist in establishing the diagnosis as well as in treating the disease. For example, the administration of glucose to a comatose patient

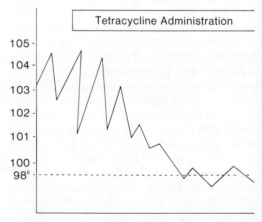

Figure 2.5. A 6-year-old child with fever and rash suggestive of Rocky Mountain spotted fever. Decrease in fever concomitant with tetracycline administration (see adjacent text for discussion).

with signs consistent with hypoglycemia may assist in establishing this metabolic state prior to the availability of confirmatory blood glucose levels. At the same time, it is curative for the disordered homeostatic state. Administration of digitalis can assist in differentiating the sometimes-confusing picture of cardiac failure from pulmonary infection. Administration of vitamin B_6 in certain convulsive disorders in some young infants may confirm the presence of the B_6-dependent seizure state. And so on.

Therapeutic trials must be undertaken judiciously. As has been discussed, they can be misleading. Further, they may complicate the clinical course of the process under investigation. A good example of this is the superimposition of drug fever in an individual to whom antibiotics have been given to help differentiate bacterial from viral etiology. The adverse reaction to the therapy in instances such as this serve to further obscure the original diagnosis as well as to create a new problem.

Testing of hypotheses does not always yield a positive result. The hypotheses may be denied, in which case alternative hypotheses must be proposed and tested. In some cases the laboratory data will suggest additional lines of historical inquiry or the necessity for more thorough and detailed examination of some part of the body. This new data collection is then blended with the previous data plus the laboratory data, new linkages are formed, and the original hypothesis is either modified or restated. An example of this can be found in the 17-year-old young man who presented with cervical adenitis and marked pharyngitis. All the evidence pointed to Group A beta-hemolytic streptococcal disease. Appropriate cultures were obtained from the throat, and his peripheral blood was examined. It was discovered that he had a high proportion of atypical lymphocytes, which led to a more careful history, which yielded that others in his group had experienced mononucleosis in recent months. Further, reexamination of his abdomen resulted in the palpation of a slightly enlarged, very "soft" spleen which had been missed initially. His throat culture yielded a Group A beta-hemolytic streptococcus. Thus the diagnosis was appropriately modified to include infectious mononucleosis and confirm the streptococcal coexistent infection.

This reexamination of data based upon additional data serves to emphasize the dynamic nature of the process of problem solving. The procedure is not so mathematical and precise that one has fixed data, rigidly structured theories and absolute proofs. Rather, the data are infinite in variety and shadings and often so subjective as to be susceptible to varied interpretations. Our hypotheses are just that, intelligent conjectures to explain the data. They should be and are fluid, subject to revision to the point of total restatement. The process is dynamic and requires constant rethinking in order to function for the patient's benefit.

CLINICAL ACTION

Apart from therapeutic tests, decisions to undertake therapy usually complete the formal problem-solving process. Often this step is viewed as a "cookbook" process. "Find the disease and look up the treatment" is an adage often echoing in medical school corridors. And often this is true—the brunt of "thinking" occurs during data collection, hypothesis formulation and testing. But not always! Even a cursory examination of most clinical situations will reveal an element of decision making. For otitis media the decision to treat is automatic, but the particular regimen chosen will depend on the age of the child, presumed etiologic agents, pharmacology of the various antibiotics, and even such mundane considerations as palatability and cost. It is not surprising that four very different regimens are chosen by thoughtful physicians.

Clinical action decisions occasionally mean *no* therapy. For example, the woman who is rubella-susceptible, becomes exposed to rubella and develops the disease in the first trimester of pregnancy incurs a risk to her unborn fetus of the congenital rubella syndrome. She and her physician can elect (1) trusting to chance (only 50% of fetuses are affected) *or* (2) undergoing therapeutic abortion. In many circumstances, abortion is unthinkable to patient and/or physician. What to do? Nothing. The physician may opt to recommend gamma globulin on the theoretic grounds that the passively acquired antibody will protect the fetus from circulating rubella virus. Scientific investigation has clearly shown that this does *not* occur—gamma globulin does not protect. The correct therapeutic problem solving is no therapy—not an ineffective one. This is a thoughtful decision utilizing the same elements as before—data, hypotheses and testing. That it is a therapeutic decision does not change the basic character of the process.

SUMMARY

In this chapter, I have attempted to give a broad overview of the major elements of clinical problem solving. In addition, I have attempted to build the philosophic framework in which this process occurs and, where appropriate, have pointed out learning cues to the student at all levels. The next several chapters will review the individual elements in greater detail, utilizing clinical examples.

Chapter 3

Data Collection

In solving clinical problems the physician uses a variety of information or data. Some information comes from the patient's voluntary expression of what he senses, feels and perceives. Some is obtained by questioning the patient to elicit nonvoluntary responses, forgotten sensations or related bits of information. Some comes from the physician's store of knowledge or from sources of information available to him. Some derives from the examination of the patient. Some derives from clinical, laboratory, radiologic or other tests.

These data do not exist in a vacuum as separate entities; they are part of a whole, and each bit represents a small portion or sample of the total information available. One of the commonest errors in medical diagnosis is to treat each symptom, sign or finding as an isolated expression having its own existence. Many errors in interpretation of clinical data stem from this oversimplification. Many individuals have been subjected to continual diagnostic testing and therapy because their concentration of hemoglobin was viewed as a single solitary fact existing in splendid isolation. The pregnant female with "anemia," the infant with "hypogamma-globulinemia," the child with some "growth disorder," the teenager with "thyroid problems," the young adult with "VD," the executive with "angina," the housewife with a "urinary tract infection" are all common ex-

amples of patients with nonexistent "diseases" which have their origin in single bits of information treated as if they were the whole individual. One of the first principles in clinical medicine is that these bits of information, clinical data, are all linked to the entire individual.

LINKAGE—THE CONCEPT OF NONISOLATION OF DATA

A hemoglobin value of 10 gm/100 ml of plasma has no meaning in itself except as an expression of a specific concentration of a single constituent of blood. It can be a normal finding in pregnancy, at certain points in infancy, and for certain patients with anemia who are recovering. It is abnormal only in reference to the individual who possesses this concentration and to specific clinical circumstances in that individual's life. It is not abnormal in itself.

This simple example is fairly clear to everyone. The same principle when applied to symptoms and signs is less apparent. A symptom may have no significance unless one considers the individual who voices it, the physiologic and psychologic state of that individual, and the specific environment in which it occurs. A "headache" of the same proportion, intensity and location in an ambitious aspiring young executive, in a housewife with 5 children, in a child of 10, and in an individual who is 85 years old does not carry the same weight or significance. In fact, unless more is known of the headache's *linkages*, one would be hard put to assign any significance to the symptom alone. By linkage I mean all those elements that influence, condition and relate to the specific bit of data.

Earlier, I referred to a 6-week-old male infant with persistent vomiting for 4 weeks. One cannot "make a diagnosis" based upon that data, but certain linkages do appear. The age and sex of the child place the vomiting in a different perspective than if we were referring to a 36-year-old woman. The persistence of the vomiting over a 4-week period changes our weighting of it. It cannot be considered trivial, it is unlikely to be due to a minor problem at this age, and its persistence suggests serious, continuing disease.

As more information is gathered, these linkages will become firmer or weaker. If a total pattern emerges, we will make a diagnosis. But before that process even begins we must establish, for each bit of information, its perspective in the individual.

Thus, great emphasis is laid upon precise data collection in medical education. We will devote the rest of this chapter to a detailed consideration of data collection and its vital role in the problem-solving process.

DATA VOLUNTEERED BY AND ELICITED FROM THE PATIENT (THE HISTORY)

A large portion of a medical history consists of volunteered statements from some informant, usually, but not always, the patient. Good data collection of this sort is an art which can be cultivated and should be. There are several "rules" to help guide us in this effort:

1. Always *gauge* the accuracy, bias and cooperation of the informant, to the extent possible.
2. Listen, listen, listen, listen.
3. Aim for precision.
4. Search for relatedness.
5. Be as complete as is necessary for both the immediate problem and the overall health of the individual.
6. Never let the problem become more important than the patient.

In what seems to be a basic contradiction, informants do not always cooperatively tell the truth or provide needed information. Although it is true that most patients want to be helped, they are not schooled in medicine and are capable of influencing the character of symptom expression because of their problems, concerns and anxieties.

To begin with, the patient usually feels, senses or perceives something wrong with his body or its functions. In medical jargon this is the chief complaint or presenting symptom. We have preached this concept for so long and so hard that it is no wonder that students become fixated upon this bit of data. However, what the patient feels, senses or perceives may be only a part of the problem or a minor component or not medically related at all. This does not diminish its importance to the patient, nor the necessity for you to pay attention to it, but it should serve to caution you from overemphasizing the role of the chief complaint. The old joke of the woman who entered the hospital with pain in her great toe and subsequently had a cholecystectomy, hysterectomy and bronchoscopy, only to be discharged in great sadness because her toe still hurt, is exemplary of this phenomenon.

To solve clinical problems, one must know what they are. The patient provides you with his recital of what his problems are; you may uncover others. In all instances they should be identified and dealt with (or not) as seems appropriate.

Patients, like people, come in different sizes, shapes and dispositions. There are those who are lucid, intelligent and cooperative; others who are less intelligent, unclear in expression, and uncooperative. And there are all shades in between. You must assess each for what he is. You won't like all of your patients, you may even "hate" some of them (e.g., the parent who abuses a child), but you are pledged to help all of them.

As a first step, learn to assess them as people and as providers of data. Your "antennae" must be tuned to others and attentive to signs of bias, prejudice, modesty, inaccuracy, loneliness and the hundreds of other human traits that will color, distort, modify, or otherwise influence a straight recital of the facts. One is reminded of the rural stereotype who enters a physician's office and responds to the question of why he is there with a stern reminder that the doctor should figure that out, that's what he's being paid for! Solid stuff for comedians but also true in the actual practice of medicine.

Let me again emphasize your role as an objective observer: Do not let your own emotions, especially those concerned with antipathy towards the patient, interfere with your help to that individual. All physicians have helped recalcitrant, hostile patients—that's what your oath is all about. In my own practice I encounter parents who physically abuse children, a condition which raises ugly emotions within me. In each instance I must place these to one side and assist that family in "solving" their problem.

The first rule then is to become an objective observer and to assign some value to the data you are collecting. Later on, as you approach analysis of the problem(s), this assessment will help guide you in weighing the significance of the data.

Of all the skills and attitudes necessary in good data collecting the most important is the ability to listen. Much important information is lost, misunderstood, incompletely collected, or misinterpreted due to defects in this trait in physicians. Example upon example can be given to illustrate the prime role of listening in data collection. It is understandable that tired, hurried, harassed physicians attempt to speed the data collection by leading their patients. Unfortunately, they may lead the patient right past the problem or into a problem that doesn't exist. Further, a patient who perceives that he is not being listened to will stop volunteering important information. Too often have we witnessed an interview which begins well and then drifts into a monosyllabic question-answer exercise. A good rule to follow is to listen to as much patient-offered information as is necessary to define the problem(s). I'm sympathetic to the physician caught with a garrulous, wandering patient, but not to the abrupt cutoff of information essential to the patient's problem.

As stated previously, data collection is an artful technique which can, and must, be acquired. No one can tell you exactly how to do this in the myriad of clinical encounters you will have. In general, each interview of other-than-an-emergency nature should begin with an opportunity for the patient to describe the problem as he sees it. As the interview progresses, the physician can adjust the pace and direction if it is too slow or too wandering. During the initial listening phase the physician can gauge his informant and get some sense of just how much direction this particular patient will need. Some require virtually none; others will only respond to a question-answer format. If all patients are given the opportunity to recite at the beginning, the interview will be more productive regardless of its final form. If you find you are impatient and tend to interject too quickly, train yourself to listen for a set period of time, during which you make a conscious effort to contain your desire for the rapid pursuit of facts.

One side effect of not listening is loss of patient confidence. Many physicians are characterized as "cold" or "scientific" or a variety of like terms simply because they fail to interact in human fashion with their patients, one component of which is listening.

Precision in data collection is similar to precision in any problem-solving situation. Can you imagine an engineer describing a bridge to be built as "about 1,000 feet long" or beams made of "metal" or the length of time to completion as "4 to 10 years?" Mathematical precision is not always possible in medical data collection, but one need not necessarily be so vague as to invalidate the effort. "Vomiting" is not precise; its type, frequency, duration, association with pain, with eating and with certain stimuli, and other characteristics make it more precise. So too with every elicited or volunteered symptom. Many texts have been written on this subject. I will not burden this chapter with aid in definition. The student will find ample sources in the references cited at the end of this text.

Precision also applies to physical findings; here the means are closer to mathematical, although not quite. One can learn to both detect and report physical findings with great precision. Thus "ulcers in the mouth" is imprecise; "3- to 5-minute shallow ulcerations on the buccal mucosa localized solely to the anterior pillars in linear array . . . etc." paints a much clearer picture of the observed lesions. A "lump in the breast" is almost meaningless in the absence of size, location, density, transillumination characteristics, mobility, adherence to other breast structure, etc.

As a group, physicians are very sloppy in their quantitative expression. Persistence of such terms as "X finger breadths" to describe organ size or extension beyond natural body boundaries is inexcusable. Whose fingers? With what relationships? A physician must learn both detection and reporting of physical findings in the most quantitative language possible. A useful guide is to consider each clinical description as a letter to some other physician who will read it 5 years from now. Will he know what you saw, heard, felt, smelled or otherwise detected? Or will he dismiss your findings as irrelevant because of vagueness and imprecision? If you apply this guideline to everything you write clinically, you will serve your patients and yourself as well as those others who must use the recorded information.

One disastrous result of a survey conducted in physician's offices by a national specialty organization was the recognition that one could not judge the adequacy of patient care by physicians' records. Their records were simply lacking in precision for all sorts of data, ranging from history through therapy and counseling. You have an opportunity to avoid this particular pitfall by establishing early in your career the habit of precise definition—in data collection and recording as well as in all aspects of the medical process.

As has been emphasized previously, individual bits of data do not exist separately. As you obtain historical information it is essential that natural relatedness of one bit to another evolves. Thus, "diarrhea" may be related to ingestion of certain foods, to activity, to environmental stimuli and to countless other factors intrinsic and extrinsic to the patient. A colleague of mine established the diagnosis in a man with a disfiguring, painful ulcerative lesion of the upper gum simply because he took the time to relate the ulceration to the individual's practice of placing aspirin tablets locally in the mouth as an analgesic. This simple association eluded primary physician and consultants alike and resulted in a protracted illness with attendant costly, elaborate and unnecessary diagnostic and therapeutic procedures. This blatant example serves as an extreme to the much more subtle failures to seek or find the relatedness of events in a patient's recital.

Some kinds of relatedness occur with such frequency that we've come to regard them as a unit: excessive thirst, hunger and urination in a diabetic; frequency of urination, dysuria and nocturia in patients with urinary tract infections; cough, hemoptysis and night sweats in cavitary pulmonary tuberculosis, and so on. Others are infrequently associated, and only careful data collection with attention to relatedness in time or process will uncover them. Some are rarely associated, and only astute perception yields detection. In all instances the relatedness must either be suggested by the patient or perceived by the physician. The individual bits of data will not just fall together; their association must be "seen" by some observer. Your antennae should always be extended in this direction, seeking those interconnections that will assist in the solution of the clinical problem.

"Thoroughness" and "completeness" are the bane of the beginning student and resident. He is expected to obtain all available information, present and past, relevant and irrelevant, medical and nonmedical, in each patient he encounters. The long "histories and physicals" of the beginning clinical clerk are like an albatross around his neck. There are several purposes of this technique of medical education. First, it will familiarize you with all components of a history. There is no substitute for personal involvement in such data collection. Second, it permits an opportunity to exercise precision in expression. Only by repetitive experience will the ability to write concisely, clearly and quantitatively come to you. Third, if diligently pursued, it will instruct you in the next process, that of condensation of information.

Not all medical encounters require the thoroughness or completeness of a beginning clinical clerk's manuscript. This is considered heresy in some circles but, in fact, is true. To solve some emergent problems, one need not obtain massive data. An example I've often used is that of the man who enters the emergency room with an ice pick projecting from his back. One does not sit down and begin an orderly process of transit from chief complaint to social history. One tends to the problem and utilizes that information essential to its complete solution. However, this does not take away from the necessity in the future of ascertaining a social profile. The latter may assist immeasurably in implementing measures to reduce the risk of a second ice pick finding its way into the same back! This lesson is lost on many physicians who, having survived the requirements of the junior clerk for lengthy "work-ups," quickly adopt a "here today, gone tomorrow" approach to medical practice. The important point is to understand the nature of the physician's obligation to his patient and to himself. He must be able to serve the patient's needs in the particular relationship he has with that patient. If he is a primary care physician, he will subserve all of the needs of the population he cares for. At some point in the relationship he will require a fairly total profile of his patient—medical, psychologic, social and economic. However, for any given phase of care he may require only a limited spectrum of information from the enormous array available for any individual. Thus, to care for a bruised knee will require less data than to care for an episode of intractable abdominal pain. The physician must cultivate the ability to adjust his data collection up and down the scale of available information. But he cannot do so unless he knows and is practical at the entire scale. One should be able to expand or contract any portion of the history at will. If a patient complains of gastrointestinal bleeding, an entire series of inquiries should follow, designed to specify, locate, relate and assess.

The final guideline is at the heart of medicine. More important than any technical skill is the ability to recognize *constantly* that it is not a fascinating problem you're confronting but a fellow human who is distressed. Many doctor-patient relationships become doctor-problem or doctor-disease relationships. Nothing will stem a patient's cooperation and confidence as being treated as an object. Most

patient dissatisfaction with physicians has its origin in the nonlistening physician who views his patients solely as possessors of the real essence of medicine, the disease.

Often this is not a blatant behavior on the part of the physician; rather, it takes the form of subtle signals. How often do we hear phrases such as "another back to see at 11" or "Mrs. Jones, you know, the one with that fascinating case of lupus" or "got to raise that hemoglobin" or countless other thoughtless, dehumanizing expressions? It is hoped that as young physicians you are motivated by humane principles. You should maintain this approach, nurture it and cultivate it through your years of learning. You should never permit the intellectual satisfaction of acquiring knowledge to replace the human elements in your relationship with patients. For those interested in efficiency, it must be restated that genuine interest in your patient will result in a more productive interview, in facilitated examination technique and in cooperation with your diagnostic and therapeutic plans.

THE PHYSICIAN'S STORE OF KNOWLEDGE AS DATA

Knowledge and a physician's command and application of it are the cornerstone of modern medical practice and problem solving. But knowledge alone is insufficient, as has been discussed in previous sections and will be taken up again. The "book" physician may be terribly knowledgeable but be unable to utilize this knowledge for his patient.

Notwithstanding this phenomenon, a physician's command of the facts of medicine is important. It is the "data" he uses to interpret and integrate data obtained from the patient. One can be a good data collector and not be able to use the data to solve the patient's problem. For example, many nurses in the past, and physician's assistants in the present, have been trained to obtain a history and perform a partial or complete physical examination. However, few are able to go much beyond this accurate recording of patient-derived data. They simply do not have the pathophysiologic understanding nor the command of an enormous body of knowledge that permits them to link together findings and pathophysiology.

The sources of information available to physicians are many and varied: (1) knowledge of anatomy, biochemistry, physiology, microbiology—the basic sciences; (2) knowledge of pharmacology and pathology—the clinicobasic sciences; (3) knowledge of clinical medicine; (4) additions to knowledge in each of these areas with the passage of time; and (5) common sense.

THE BASIC SCIENCES

Many students bemoan the beginning years of medical school. Typical comments include, "it's too basic," "it has nothing to do with clinical medicine," "it's boring," "it's only research-oriented," and so on. All of these comments are wrong, as evidenced by the more mature student's attitude which reflects the appreciation of the framework of medical knowledge. Senior students come to appreciate the interrelationships between the basic fund of biomedical knowledge and clinical application. Often for the first time they sense that disease processes and molecular biology are really the same thing. How often has a senior student yearned to return to his basic science education because of this fresh perception of its value? Modern medical curricula have acknowledged this phasing of appreciation and perception by allowing liberal elective time towards the end of medical school to permit "return to the basics."

A physician is a poor doctor if he does not have in his immediate recall useful anatomic, physiologic and biochemical principles. He may be baffled by the new antibiotic or the new vaccine if he doesn't understand basic microbiology. These are not anachronistic studies for the beginning medical student. They are solid foundation on which he will build his own personal fund of knowledge. Intracellular organization, electron transport, contractility of muscle, and phage replication in bacteria, all seem abstract and in a world divorced from medicine. Yet each of these concepts is ensconced solidly in today's clinical practice and promises to become instrumental in new modes of therapy and diagnosis. There is no substitute for a good solid underpinning of basic science information.

THE CLINICOBASIC SCIENCES

Pharmacology and pathology are natural links between classic basic science disciplines and clinical medicine. Both blend basic molecular biologic knowledge with applicability to a greater degree than most disciplines. Most importantly, both contain knowledge that the clinician will use daily for the rest of his professional life.

The study of pharmacology should set out for the student those concepts concerning chemical and other modes of therapy upon which he will base future therapeutic decisions. If he understands the adrenergic receptor system and the principle of beta-blockade, an entire array of therapeutic variations in allergy, hypertension, shock, etc. are instantly available to him. If he grasps the mechanism and expression of untoward reactions to drugs, he will not be mystified by drug fever, allergic reactions, hematopoietic effects and other important clinical manifestations of drug use. Today's medicine is in large measure the correct therapeutic application of an entire array of chemical agents which interact with human or microbial metabolic systems to produce desired effects. One can easily become a "pill pusher" with no real knowledge of these potent agents, or one can benefit his patients by the thoughtful choice and application of appropriate drugs. The study of pharmacology is the keystone to correct, judicious and wise use of these potent agents.

Pathology is the hub of clinical medicine. Virtually every organic disorder and some psychiatric ones have origins in known pathologic processes. Even if our knowledge of the etiology of a given disease is muddy and uncertain, certain pathologic information is available. More than any other body of knowledge, pathology is of greatest aid to clinical problem solving. Our ability to link and integrate patient-derived data is founded in a keen appreciation of pathophysiologic changes. Jaundice as a symptom achieves its diagnostic significance to us by virtue of our understanding of those aspects of production, metabolism and excretion of bilirubin in relation to the tissues and organs involved. Knowledge of pathology allows orchestration of anatomic, metabolic and physiologic information. It permits us to hold a framework against which the data available to us can be cast. The pattern, form and substance of the resulting analysis allows for problem solving.

It is not by chance that the study of pathology usually sits astride the basic science of clinical curricula. It is the link, and a good clinician or diagnostician is good by virtue of his appreciation for, and application of, pathologic fact and principle.

KNOWLEDGE OF CLINICAL MEDICINE

Clinical knowledge is an elusive substance—difficult to define and essential to have. When one refers to a doctor as a good clinician or diagnostician, one usually means that in that individual is blended skill, art and knowledge. The clinical knowledge component is composed of a sound base in molecular biologic knowledge, an understanding of how normal becomes abnormal and an appreciation of the variations of expression of abnormality. The formal study of clinical medicine has become discipline-oriented, but the true body of knowledge cuts across all disciplines.

One really doesn't have pediatric, obstetric or psychiatric knowledge; rather, one has applied general medical concepts to a specific population or specific area of pathophysiology. Excellence in any discipline is the hallmark of command of general medical principles. One sees this evident in those areas that blend disciplines—adolescent medicine (internal medicine, pediatrics, psychiatry, gynecology), perinatal medicine (neonatology, obstetrics), psychosomatic disease (internal medicine, psychiatry) and others. In these areas adjacent to more than one discipline, the basic clinical knowledge also becomes blended, and information is less discipline-oriented than general medicine-oriented. This point is often lost on the student who sees knowledge arrayed by clinical service or by the textbook of X or by rigidly designed clinical units which separate a given category of patient. However, jaundice in the newborn, the child, the adolescent or the adult is dependent upon the same mechanisms, given variation for maturity and structure. Problem solving in the jaundiced patient does not confine itself to the discipline that has segregated the patient. The process is identical in each discipline; what varies is slight population-oriented differences in pathophysiology.

Clinical knowledge then is an extension of basic science and clinicobasic science information heavily rooted in pathophysiology and adorned with specific data concerning clinical expression. That our art or science is not a rigidly defined body of knowledge is evident most visibly in the clinical arena. Here one must learn the nuances of subjectivity of facts, the factor of experience, and the value of personal sensory perception in shaping clinical knowledge. We simply do not know everything there is to know about medicine. The degree to which we understand variation in human expression of pathophysiology is the degree to which we are knowledgeable. Sir William Osler, an outstanding clinician in medicine, has left a legacy of clinical aphorisms. One of these pithy comments is:

> "Variability is the law of life, and as no two faces are the same, so no two bodies are alike, and no two individuals react alike and behave alike under the abnormal conditions which we know as disease."

An example might illustrate and clarify this point. Typhoid fever typically is a septic disease *without* initial gastrointestinal manifestations; i.e., there is no diarrhea. Almost all textbooks cite this "fact," teachers teach it, and students learn it. What of the following case, then?

> A 17-year-old male presented following 2 days of severe diarrhea, developed a fever of septic type ranging from 101° to 105° F. In the ensuing week he developed lethargy, profound anorexia and complained constantly of pain in various parts of the body. A generalized headache with localization to his forehead was cited, and he also had a nonproductive, persistent cough. At this point *Salmonella typhi* was grown from his blood and bone marrow specimens.

The clinician was confronted with an "atypical" syndrome with many classic features of typhoid fever but with the presence of diarrhea. He correctly interpreted this as a probable instance of typhoid fever despite the diarrhea and established the diagnosis by appropriate cultures. Subsequent information indicated a particularly heavy source of contamination, the ingestion of a large quantity of infected, partially cooked turkey. Under these circumstances diarrhea can occur.

Clinical knowledge in this case consisted of retention and recall on the physician's part of the typical and usual typhoid manifestations. The unusual features are not in store of knowledge of most physicians but did not deter this particular clinician in this situation.

It is instances such as this one which underscore the vast range of information available, the imperfection of absolute knowledge, and the variability of expression of disease. These factors make clinical knowledge an ill-defined entity which in contradictory fashion must, nonetheless, be learned. The beginning student is often overwhelmed by these considerations; he must remember constantly that to learn to run, one must first crawl and then walk.

Acquisition of clinical knowledge is a continuous, lifelong process. One must only look as far as the most recent journals to appreciate the constant modification, addition and elaboration of current knowledge. This is such an important phenomenon we will consider it separately and more fully.

CONTINUING EDUCATION

Continuing education is the addition to, modification of and elaboration upon a basic store of information.

At one time it was possible for an individual to become learned in medicine as a result of 4 years of medical school and appropriate postgraduate training in his chosen discipline. Since the late 1940's and early 1950's this is no longer possible. One never achieves total knowledge in any area of medicine in a lifetime. Rather, one achieves a basic framework to the discipline of medicine during his medical school days, embellishes this with the experience of a residency, and continues to learn thereafter.

Medical school education usually provides a sound base, but the necessity and techniques for future learning are insufficiently stressed. Most physicians discover this later in their careers when implementation of learning techniques may be made more dif-

ficult by the exigencies of daily practice and living. *It is imperative for every student of medicine and resident physician to develop the techniques and habits of constant learning early in his education.*

What are the sources and methods usually employed in continuing education, the term given to the process of acquisition of new information, of modifying old concepts and facts, and of elaboration of principles and data?

These are listed in Table 3.1 and considered in more detail here.

Peer contact is a time-honored method for improving one's knowledge. Medicine retains some characteristics of the heritage of apprenticeship which is rooted in its early origins. Throughout medical education one learns from those above him on the knowledge-experience hierarchy scale. This tradition is firmly established in our educational system. Physicians can derive much direct information and indirect leads to new information from productive contact with peers. These contacts range from informal, chance encounters to highly structured meetings of various types.

One group practice in my region utilizes a weekly "journal" club which is designed to utilize all information a single individual acquires from whatever source for the group's benefit. Meetings attended, books read, journal articles analyzed, a good audiotape, etc. are presented and discussed. In this way, members of this group keep abreast of changes in medical knowledge. Singular, sig-

Table 3.1
Sources of Continuing Education

Peer contact
Conferences and seminars
   Local
   Regional
   National
Textbooks
Medical magazines and throwaways
Audiovisual devices
   Educational
   Commercial
Journals
Drug literature and inserts
Detail man and advertising
Others

nificant advances can be highlighted at this meeting and subsequently explained in depth by those to whom it has been exposed. One cannot underestimate this source as a means of expanding one's horizons.

Another form of peer contact of especial value is that afforded by consultation. The consultant is usually well versed in an area of medicine with which the physician has minimal or incomplete contact. This provides an opportunity stemming from a specific patient encounter to be expanded to an educational experience.

A second source of information is the more formal conference. I use this term in a generic sense for all gatherings in which a single physician is seeking information in a structured setting. Depending on locale, these conferences may take the form of patient-oriented discussions (case conferences, "grand" rounds, peer review meetings, clinicopathologic presentations, etc.) or topic-oriented lectures or discussion. They are invaluable to all physicians at one time or another and to some physicians as the most efficient method for them to learn.

Conferences occur at the local level in hospitals, group practices, medical societies, special-interest clubs, and medical schools and by invited "foreigners"—variations upon the visiting professorship. They can take place at the state or regional level, in which case they are mostly topic-oriented and broader in scope than most local conferences. Or they can occur as national meetings, usually associated with an individual's chosen discipline. National meetings tend to be topic-oriented with focus upon many topics in a given year, usually selected because of current interest or for reasons of continuing importance to that discipline.

The standard fare of medical students, the textbook, assumes less importance in continuing education. However, it is a neglected personal source from which many physicians could easily benefit. The textbook is always available, can be as personalized as one wishes to the point of writing in it, and provides someone's organization of medical knowledge in the area it covers. The disadvantage of this source is the necessary delay in publication which renders some of the information "old" or inapplicable. This factor has been overstated by zealots. Most material in textbooks *is* usable and correct and true. Not all knowledge is in constant revolutionary upheaval, and one can learn a great deal from standard textbook content. A more serious disadvantage is the restricted viewpoint that some textbooks provide. Subject to an author's variability and inadequacies, to editorial needs for brevity, and to other factors, textbooks may present a highly stilted or stunted version of the "truth." Viewpoints which are at variance with the author's or editor's may be omitted or presented in an unfavorable light. Discussion in depth may be precluded. Oversimplification may be presented as the total picture for a complex, convoluted issue. Selection of subtopics may be limited, and the precise information you seek and need may not be there. Difficult questions arising in clinical practice may not be represented. And finally, the facts may be wrong. Our society has come to so revere the printed word that what is stated in medical textbooks is often taken as the gospel. It may, in fact, be a distortion, an untruth, a misunderstanding or a highly biased interpretation.

Notwithstanding all objections to the use of textbooks, they do provide an avenue of information acquisition that is convenient and personal. To some physicians and for some areas of medical knowledge there is no good substitute for an authoritative textbook.

Today's physician is deluged with what is probably the least valuable form of continuing education—the medical magazine and throwaway.

This bold and all-encompassing statement, as for most of its nature, needs some modification. There are *good* magazines and throwaways, and there is some good information in most. But the gold among the dross is difficult to see and, to the uncritical reader, impossible to distinguish. Commercial interests understand the enormous need of physicians to be constantly reevaluating themselves and have seized upon the capsule presentation as an effective service. In so doing, the material presented is often sensationalized, made superficial, oversimplified, presented as fact when it is conjecture, presented as the accomplished, final and definitive products of investigation when it is preliminary, pilot or sketchy in origin, and offered in such glib language as to convince the reader of its merit.

If all of the magazines and throwaways were to disappear instantly, we would lose a few sources of solid continuing education, but for the most part we would have lost nothing. You cannot be educated in a reliable, consistent fashion by a diet consisting solely of such fare. Given limited time and opportunity for medical reading, you are well advised to discard such junk mail in preference for textbook and journal reading.

To some physicians, learning is more readily accomplished by the spoken word rather than by reading. For these individuals there is a plethora of taped programs available which have some positive and some negative aspects.

Commending this approach to continuing education is the utility of this audio source of information. The busy physician can listen to these tapes while engaged in other activities, such as driving to and from the office or hospital or during physical exercises. They have the advantage of currency—the tapes are produced quickly and distributed rapidly after production, so the information gap secondary to time is minimized. They employ experts, and thus the information is frequently very valuable and to the point. Lastly they are brief and concise, allowing increments of knowledge which most people can absorb easily.

The disadvantages include all of the plagues of textbook production: selectivity of topic and expert; editorial considerations; the necessity for clear exposition as well as a good speaking voice, not necessarily coincident with expertise; and the expense, which can be considerable when compared to other sources.

More recently the "visual" has been added to the audio, and we now have a plethora of relatively easily played videotapes. This technique combines the advantages of listening with the display of various kinds of visual material. At its best it can enhance learning and augment description with invaluable illustration—the "picture is worth 10,000 words" phenomenon. At its worst it can be sloppily constructed, with poor or inaccurate visuals.

Physicians find it difficult to utilize journal reading for a variety of reasons, most remediable. First, many leave medical school with only a scant appreciation of this source of information, its value and validity. Second, few have cultivated the necessary discipline and habit required to read regularly and critically. As the "business" of medical practice increases and time restraints become real, few will read regularly unless they have already established a pattern. My own suggestion to students is to begin reading general medical journals, such as the *New England Journal of Medicine*, the *Journal of the American Medical Association*, *Lancet* or many others, early in their clinical education. The student should discipline himself to read these regularly appearing periodicals prior to the next edition. Regardless of other activities, some time should be set aside devoted exclusively to the dissection of the journals. At the beginning the array of articles will be overwhelming. At this point the student should begin the process of selective reading. Articles of general medical interest should be read in their entirety. Features such as clinicopathologic conferences or summary articles on new advances should likewise be read as a whole. Other articles and features should be scanned, and still others only superficially examined. The student should use his developing interests to guide him in this selectivity. It does not matter what he reads at this point, only that he reads regularly and begins critical analysis. As he explores each discipline in the usual rotations he should sample the available literature. Some disciplines will assist him by assignment of expectation; in others he will have to seek faculty advice on what there is and what he should be reading. As his career interests become more focal he should begin to include major journals in that field in his regular habit, so that upon entering a residency he will be able to continue his regularity. At this point he will become highly selective in the journals he reads but still be exploratory and probing in the specific articles and features he distributes among the categories of completeness in reading. From this point on, his focus will be individual, and just what and how much of what he reads will be determined by his own needs and interests.

By utilizing available journal articles and other sources (peers, faculty), he will develop the art of critical reading. The printed word will not always be chapter and verse; rather, he will learn the value of judgement as to an author's methods and conclusions.

By carrying over into practice the regularity of the habit of reading journals and cultivating criticality, he has the essential tools of continuing education in his own hands and under control.

Another source of difficulty in achieving consistent journal reading is the content of many journals. They may emphasize what to the physician is trivia or minutia when measured against the yardstick of practice needs. One cannot discuss this situation adequately except in terms of specific journals and specific content. However, some general principles emerge. Each discipline has an array of journals. By selecting those among the multitude that suit your needs, you may be able to overcome this difficulty. Also, one finds that even in journals not thought to contain needed information are articles and sections which are valuable. Again, one must approach the specific journal not as something to be ingested *in toto* but as a smorgasbord of information, some of which is sampled, some of which is ignored, and some of which is selected for the main course.

I cannot overemphasize the care with which consistent, valuable reading is established by the early institution of discipline and the sequential acquisition of critical analysis. Nor can the difficulty of continuing education be overemphasized in the absence of such discipline. It is as important for the student to establish this habit as it is for him to learn the basics. The basics he learns today will be modified with time, and only by reading can he adequately "keep up" with the transition.

Another source of information proving to be of increasing value to the clinician is drug information. Today this takes the form of literature distributed by manufacturers and of inserts necessary in each package of a given medication. In addition, interested but unbiased experts have put together various kinds of summary evaluations of new drugs (e.g., *Medical Letter*). The modern regulatory climate has forced the inclusion of data on efficacy, pharmacology and toxicity in these kinds of drug information. A wise physician will read the material on a new medication *prior to* administering it to a single patient. He will also search out and read evaluations of such therapy in his regularly read journals and textbooks.

The least effective way to learn about drugs is from so-called "detail men" or from advertising. It is understandable that the virtues of a given preparation will be extolled and the disadvantages or adverse effects soft-pedaled or even ignored. This does not excuse the clinician from relying solely on this source of information. He would be very foolish to restrict his education to such biased sources. This does not mean that the "detail" approach is without merit or that advertising is totally misleading. Both can yield valuable information in quick fashion, but such information will most likely be incomplete.

There are other sources of continuing education beyond the scope of this discussion.

In summary, the good physician will utilize a variety of sources to amend his already substantial fund of knowledge. He does so with the understanding that in order to solve clinical problems in his patients, he needs to place patient-derived data into a perspective of disease which will enable him to reach satisfactory diagnostic conclusions. He knows that he cannot do so on an inadequate supply of information. If he does not continue his education beyond its initial phases, he will be unprepared for the challenges of clinical medicine in his lifetime.

COMMON SENSE

Medical knowledge is often treated as an entity entirely separate from other human endeavor. This is an erroneous concept. A physician must be generally knowledgeable concerning the world about him; he must have common sense. Pure application of medical concepts to a specific problem often results in an overall inadequate patient outcome. Puzzled by this turn of events, many physicians fail to comprehend that the solution they offered, pure and correct as it was in medical terms, was inadequate for the patient's life-style, economics or understanding. Nowhere is this more evident than in therapeutic compliance, when sensible recommendations (to the physician) are totally out of line with the patient's ability to carry them out; i.e., they are not sensible to the patient. For example, I might discover an allergic cause to a given child's repetitive severe bronchopneumonia. I can prescribe an allergen-free environment, only to have none of my recommendations carried out because they cannot be. The family cannot give a single room to the child, they live in a two-bedroom house which must accommodate both parents and four children. They cannot replace the woolens with cotton or purchase plastic covers for the bed and pillow—father doesn't earn enough. And so on. My conclusion as to therapy was correct, but I displayed little common sense in recommending it.

Similarly, patients fail to take a medication for the prescribed length of time or do not obtain needed diagnostic tests or resist necessary hospitalization because the recommendation is beyond their means of understanding. A physician with common sense will appreciate these phenomena and seek alternative solutions or special assistance to carry out his recommended program.

No one can teach common sense, and reams of discussion would not apply it to you. Only a perception on your part that you are applying the problem-solving process to a real patient in a real world will insure appropriate application. Keep your eyes and ears open and your interpersonal antennae extended for information, attitudes and conditions which will alter your final dispensation.

DATA DERIVED FROM PHYSICAL EXAMINATION*

The physical examination is an organized search for data. Many of the considerations applicable here have already been discussed under the headings of patient-derived historical data. There are some unique features of this process of data acquisition.

---

* For an excellent pediatric source, see: Barnes, LA: *Manual of Pediatric Physical Diagnosis*, 5th ed. Year Book Medical Publishers, Chicago, 1980.

The examination of the human body is limited in scope by currently available technology, by our understanding of pathophysiology, by the patient's attitudes and by the natural restrictions of our senses. In this process the physician samples cells, tissues and organs for their integrity and function. He is aware of the usual range of variability, although he continues to be surprised by those normal findings several standard deviations from the mean.

This is a highly personal process to physician and patient. Personal to the physician because it relies upon his innate and trained sensory modalities and thus varies somewhat from examiner to examiner. Personal to the patient because the object of the search, his body, is most often viewed as a private and mysterious domain. Opening it up to the impersonal probings of another involves a degree of surrender of self which may not be appreciated by the examiner. Many individuals dislike or, frankly, are repelled by the necessity to disrobe. Others resent the discomfort they associate with various maneuvers. Some are suspicious of the necessity for examination and consider it an unnecessary retreat. "After all, can't you tell what's wrong with me from the way I feel" is a commonly felt and occasionally voiced sentiment. Some have gone to great pains to provide an "image" by the clothing they wear and thus feel exposed when their bodies are viewed without the protective image shield. To the mechanical observer these feelings and sentiments are trivial and are ignored. Little wonder that the confidence of patients is shaken and their cooperation withheld.

The astute and sensitive physician must assess these feelings and modify his technique accordingly. There are many satisfactory methods for obtaining complete, reliable examination without the direct, impersonal violation of a person's dignity. Learn them and apply them to your patient encounters.

Cultivation of our manual skills is not only possible but essential. One must learn to direct his senses in such a way that they capture the information we need quickly, reliably and accurately. From the first tentative probings of our finger tips on the abdomen of our classmates in a physical diagnosis exercise to the swift, sure palpation of our 1,000th or 10,000th patient examined is a process of repetition, experience and training. In some disciplines and in most disciplines at some time, rapid acquisition of data is not only mandatory but all that can be done. Only the exercised hand and fingers, the trained eye, the keen ear and, on occasion, the sensitive nose will suffice in such circumstances.

The technique of examination, although highly structured and formalized, lends itself to considerable flexibility. Thus one can examine a 2-lb infant, a 9-month-pregnant multiparous woman and a 300-lb adult with equal competence if he employs some variations to a common theme. The student should learn not only the basic skills and techniques but also the variations and adaptations. Details of the precise methods are found in other textbooks and will not be detailed here (see "Bibliography").

The data obtained by physical examination are vital to the diagnostic or problem-solving process. Therefore, they must be precise and accurate and in a form that is usable. Much of this has been covered previously. In addition to these points one should remember that the quality of problem solving bears a direct relation to the quality of the data employed. If one detects an enlarged spleen in a patient, this has considerable significance. However, if the finding is uncertain or, worse, mistaken, all subsequent reasoning becomes indefinite or erroneous.

Another value to precision is found in continuous care and evaluation. The process of detection and recording of findings that are accurate and precise lends itself to continuous observation of change during the course of an illness. Some findings are valuable in following acute, short-term illnesses which are responding (or not) to therapy. Others will be of value in gauging the long-term course of chronic illnesses. Sloppily performed and/or recorded examination may render judgements concerning efficacy of therapy or course of disease impossible.

DATA DERIVED FROM TESTING OF HYPOTHESIS—LABORATORY, ROENTGENOLOGIC AND OTHER DATA

At once a boon to the modern physician as well as one of his most serious public liabilities, the testing of hypotheses offers a good opportunity to judge the wisdom of the clinician. There are many approaches to testing of an hypothesis, but none serves as well as that which is directed to answering specific questions. If clinical data suggest anemia, certain laboratory tests, performed in sequence, can quickly answer specific questions, such as type, extent and even cause of the anemia. On the other hand, the indiscriminate employment of a "routine" battery of tests most often will squander the patient's resources, provide reams of unwanted and unnecessary data, and on occasion will create nondisease. This point has been more fully discussed elsewhere.

In assisting the problem-solving process, laboratory data should fulfill the following criteria:

1. It should always be obtained in answer to a specific question. For each bit of laboratory data the clinician should be able to provide a clear justification rooted in the clinical data.
2. It should be as directed as is necessary. If one is following the course of disease in a given patient, one or two tests may be sufficient, rather than an entire battery yielding repetitive costly information.
3. It should be reliable. Although not always in the physician's control, the laboratory used should be the best available, with results that one can depend upon. The use of laboratories which do not have this sort of confidence can only cloud the diagnostic process at best and lead to costly and potentially dangerous diagnostic pursuit at worst.
4. It should always be integrated with clinical data. This is an exceedingly tricky area. If laboratory data do not agree with your clinical assessment of the problem, there are two major possible explanations: first, you may be correct and the result is in error; and second, your assessment may be incorrect and the laboratory's correct.

Some examples might clarify Point 4.

A 6-year-old male entered the hospital with the classic syndrome of neutrophile dysfunction—the so-called chronic granulomatous disease. Every clinical clue pointed to a defect in the white blood cells. Indeed, the laboratory confirmed this but also reported very low serum immunoglobulins, the opposite of the usual condition associated with neutrophile dysfunction. The clinician could not accept this result and reordered the test with the same result. He then paid attention to the finding and subsequently discovered a new immunologic defect not previously described.

This example points out two processes: first, the initial questioning of an unexpected result with repetition of the test; and second, the acceptance of initial error in reasoning, rethinking, and a new conclusion. At all times the clinician must be prepared to regard laboratory data in this light.

A 16-year-old female was seen because she was nervous, ate excessively, sweated profusely and felt warm all the time. Despite her numerous symptoms the physical examination revealed nothing abnormal. In testing his hypotheses the physician ordered a protein-bound iodine (PBI) level to assess thyroid function. It was high. At this point he reassessed the patient and again found nothing abnormal. He rejected the significance of the result in light of his clinical data and refused to make a diagnosis of hyperthyroidism. Subsequent history established the formerly concealed fact that large quantities of an iodine-containing "tonic" had been ingested, explaining the high PBI in the absence of clinical evidence of hyperthyroidism.

In this instance, had the clinician blindly accepted the laboratory result, he could have created a two-headed monster. First, he would have labeled this young lady with a disease she did not possess with all the psychologic implications that accompany such labeling. Second, he may have employed potent therapy to relieve her "hyperthyroid" state, creating new diseases in a physically normal young lady. In addition, he would have avoided making the correct diagnosis of anxiety neurosis and delayed appropriate psychiatric therapy.

Laboratory tests should be your servants, not your master. Too often in medical practice the results of laboratory determinations are treated as absolutes. They guide the clinician rather than the other way around. There is something magical about a printed result, and when it takes the modern form of a computer print-out, it often achieves a mystical status. Laboratory results are simply expressions of a sampling the clinician has taken of his patient's anatomy, physiology or biochemistry. They are impartial and, assum-

ing accuracy, simply record a quantitative sounding at a given point in time. They should not be regarded in any other way.

One caveat about "routines" or "batteries" as applied to laboratory testing: There is a growing sentiment in this country that good medical practice should include an instantaneous sampling of a variety of bodily functions. Thus we have routine admission "chemical profiles" and multiphasic screening batteries of tests among other random searches for data. For some clinical phenomena this idea makes sense. Mass screening for hypertension, anemia, urinary tract infections, metabolic defects and diabetes have been employed successfully. Silent diseases (without symptoms that bring patients into the health care system) can be detected in early stages. There is little quarrel with this approach, provided one recalls that not all such testing is benign. Many mistakes are made in both directions. Some disease is missed due to the insensitivity of tests employed or to errors. Some patients are incorrectly labeled with a disease or condition they do not have because the tests employed are too sensitive or mistakes are made. To assess any screening procedure, one must know the false positives and false negatives that occur.

The same principles apply to the use of "batteries" or "routines" in individual patients. A current vogue is to do and report 6 to 50 chemical and hematologic tests for each patient on admission to the hospital. The disadvantages of this method have been discussed more fully elsewhere in the text. One major negative feature is that the tests are not being applied in answer to a specific question. Thus the result one gets exists in a vacuum. The tendency to treat such results as *the* focal point for beginning the problem-solving process has inherent dangers. If, instead, the results are used to indicate clinical areas for additional probing, some justification for their use may be found. Advocates of multi-test probing imply that this is a timesaving device cutting short the days of hospitalization *because the clinician doesn't have to think*! Apparently, thinking and the time it takes is abhorent to some who would rather substitute the automated laboratory analyzer. An example follows which illustrates the worst outcome of such a mindless procedure.

During a hospitalization for moderate bronchopneumonia, a 4-year-old boy had his serum analyzed "routinely" for 12 components, including alkaline phosphatase. The laboratory data returned to the ward with conveniently shaded normal areas for each of the tests performed, with this boy's results overprinted. His alkaline phosphatase level was well above the shaded normal zone. This led his physician to order a series of specific chemical tests, several roentgenologic studies of his bones, and a consultation with an expert in metabolic diseases. Upon completion of this series of examinations which consumed several extra hospital days and considerable dollars, it was decided he was normal. Then the discovery was made that the normal zone for alkaline phosphatase was for adults and that growing children normally had levels far above adult values.

It could be argued that the above incident is not a fault of the multitest system, just a defect in the mode of reporting which is easily convertible. But why was an alkaline phosphatase determination obtained? Except for acute obstructive liver disease, a rarity in children, there is no justification for performing it at all. It is a test without a reasonable question. *Any* result is unnecessary, and errors can and do occur in both the determination and interpretation. Why should any clinician deal with totally unnecessary data and then have to explain an abnormal or apparently abnormal result? It is mindless medicine and should be avoided. Clearly, routines and batteries should be applied to a patient or a population which has a high incidence for a disease or condition the tests reflect. The entire premise of this book and the subject it treats, problem solving, is based upon the fact that there are a set of stimuli from the patient which form a problem. Obtaining unnecessary laboratory data provide indeterminate data for which there is not a corresponding problem and may lead to search for additional unnecessary data.

This discussion should not be interpreted to mean that all "battery" testing is inappropriate. Some is well founded in clinical fact and has clearly stated problems. For example, in the 1980's it is important to seek and find silent syphilis among our older child and young adult population. The routine employment of a standard screening test for syphilis is justified because it provides an answer to the simple clinical problem: Does this patient have silent syphilis? However, even with this justifiable and reasonable screening one will uncover biologic false positive reactions. Blind acceptance of the laboratory result will inevitably lead to incorrect diagnosis and a series of investigations which not only are unnecessary but may be socially stigmatizing.

The best guideline in the obtaining and interpreting of laboratory tests is that the clinician be constantly thinking—thinking about the reason for obtaining the test and thinking about the significance of the result for his patient.

SUMMARY

This chapter has dealt with the kinds of data clinicians use in problem solving. A crude classification has been developed, and definition of each type of data has been presented. The usefulness of the data and some general guidelines for obtaining and interpreting them have been presented. No problem can be solved without data; the solution will only be as good as the data that led to it.

Chapter 4

Establishing Clinical Hypotheses

INTRODUCTION

As the clinician accumulates data relevant to a specific problem posed by a patient's symptoms, he must place the information into a harmonious whole. He does so by establishing possible explanations for the patient's problems. These explanations are *hypotheses*. The development of hypotheses distinguishes the problem-solving processes from mere data collection. For example, it is possible to structure the development of historical and physical examination data into an highly organized process. Many physicians and clinics employ such data collection techniques prior to direct physician involvement. They do so by a variety of methods: computerized history, trained ancillary medical personnel, and segmented physical examination among other techniques. The collected information is of little value in itself; it simply represents bits of information, both subjective and objective, each of which is a sample of the patient's biomedical and psychologic function.

At this point a physician, or delegated person or process, must attempt to explain the pattern that the data reveal. Our discussion will be confined to the physician, and other methods will be referred to at the end of this chapter.

The physician does not establish hypotheses in a random fashion. The determinants utilized in hypothesis setting are as follows: (1) the total knowledge of the problem solver; (2) the degree to which given diseases or conditions are understood; (3) the ability of the problem solver to discern patterns, to match discerned patterns with known configurations of disease and to think logically; and (4) a set of principles which usually operates in human pathophysiology. The principles mentioned in Point 4 above are:

1. Common diseases and conditions occur commonly.
2. A single process should be invoked to explain most of the data, if not all of it.
3. Simple problems usually have simple explanations.
4. Hypotheses should derive from the data and not be imposed upon them.
5. The hypothesis should be consistent with known pathophysiologic mechanisms
6. Usually many hypotheses are developed, even if only transiently. Serious consideration of an individual hypothesis is based upon its probability.
7. Hypotheses may be formulated at any point in the diagnostic process; they may be accepted, rejected or modified during the course of problem solving.

General Considerations

In establishing hypotheses, physicians do not always consciously carry out each step. To the initiate the process may appear almost mystic or, at the very least, inspirational. Students frequently consider expert diagnosticians as paragons and are puzzled by their ability to seemingly "leap" from data to hypothesis. Despite the inability, in a specific instance, to detail each step of the problem-solving process, such steps do exist. The purpose of the discussion in this chapter is to dissect the process of establishing hypotheses in order to clarify the steps between data and action.

THE BODY OF KNOWLEDGE AND THE PHYSICIAN'S PERCEPTION OF IT

The first two factors that determine an individual's ability to establish hypotheses are concerned with knowledge. In the sense used here, knowledge means what is known about disease, both by medicine-at-large and by an individual physician. This point will not be belabored here, as it is adequately covered elsewhere in Chapter 3.

Briefly stated, hypotheses cannot be adequately established unless there is reasonable appreciation of the current universe of medical knowledge. The beginning of the problem-solving process is vested in such knowledge. It should also be obvious that the reason an hypothesis cannot be automatically set following collection of data is that medical knowledge is imperfect.

For diseases in which the manifestations are few and fairly characteristic of those diseases, the establishment of hypotheses is fairly straightforward. For example, abscesses in the distal fascial spaces, so-called "felons," present little problem to the physician. The symptoms and findings are few, very specific and very obvious to patient and physician. Establishing an hypothesis of "infection in the fascial spaces of the X distal digit" is usually simple; the only problem to be resolved is etiology. In contrast, intra-abdominal abscesses may present with a variety of symptoms, many of which are not specific. Individuals with intra-abdominal abscesses may complain of varying symptoms which can be arranged in many patterns. In these instances, many hypotheses may have to be considered.

In addition to the totality of knowledge of disease, the individual physician's appreciation of this knowledge is critical to establishing hypotheses. The greater his grasp of such medical knowledge as exists, the greater his ability to establish appropriate hypotheses. This is an obvious statement discussed in Chapter 3.

INDIVIDUAL LOGICAL ABILITY

Discussed later in this chapter, the third factor, logical thinking, is obvious. Less obvious than general logical ability is the pattern-discrimination component. Data presented by and obtained from the patient have no intrinsic configuration. It is true that certain symptoms or findings occur in groups for many diseases. But the "grouping" is usually in the eyes of the observer. An example may help to clarify this concept:

A 6-year-old female presented with intermittent abdominal pain for 3 months. The pain was usually mild, lasting from 3 to 12 hours, and localized to the umbilicus. Her physician had examined her on several occasions with an essentially negative examination except for minimal periumbilical and epigastric tenderness. Between episodes she was completely normal.

The current episode was much more severe, with recurring pain for the past 24 hours. Her mother had observed a bloody mucoid stool, which prompted her to seek medical attention. Examination reveals a blonde 6 year old who is in obvious distress, has many freckles on her face including circular brownish macules on her lips and anterior buccal mucosa. She is very fair-skinned, tans easily on exposure to the sun and currently has peeling skin on her face, neck, shoulders and extremities. Her abdomen is quiet, not distended, and with a normal percussion note throughout. Minimal tenderness is demonstrable by grimace and voluntary guarding upon deep palpation in her upper abdomen. There is no rebound, no costovertebral angle tenderness or suprapubic tenderness. Her genitalia are normal and rectal examination normal except for the presence of a small amount of muco-sanguineous fecal material on the examining finger after withdrawal.

This child has an unusual syndrome. Recognition of the *pattern* of findings is a prerequisite to diagnosis. Omitted from the description above is the myriad of normal historical and physical examination data. Can the pattern be discerned from among the almost infinite positive and negative data? It will be obvious that the patient manifests a characteristic pattern, but it is submerged in normal and nonrelated data. She suffers from the Peutz-Jeghers syndrome, consisting of intestinal polyps (hamartomas) associated with mucosal pigmentation. Her symptoms result from erosion of the polyps and/or abnormal motility of the intestine which can lead to intussusception. The grouping of findings is there but must be *observed* as a group. Negative discrimination must also occur; the sunburned skin is unrelated and does not belong in the "group" of findings.

Much of medicine consists of pattern recognition. There appears to be a specific ability, varying among individuals, to discern patterns among individual data arranged in various configurations. Most of us are familiar with visual pattern recognition in which figures, numerals or other coherent patterns are discerned against a confusing, nonorganized background. Most of us recognize the ability of some individuals to discern auditory patterns (e.g., a musical melody played against a noisy background). Less well known is the ability to assemble logical relationships from data presented as if randomly arrayed. This ability does exist and is measurable to some extent. Varying as it does among physicians, it is not surprising that some individuals more readily "grasp" such groupings of clinical data. This is a skill which can be developed or accentuated. Pattern recognition in medicine results from a learning focus upon known disease patterns on the one hand, and experiential emphasis upon groups of findings in patients, on the other hand. That is, we learn what the patterns are that we know about and how to search for them in problems presented by patients. Finally, repetition (experience) in a selected area of medicine enables the physician to increase his skills in this area. The student and resident are advised to pursue these two avenues throughout their medical education: (1) learn as much as is possible about the usual patterns of findings and (2) look for grouped findings in each patient. Further augmentation of this skill can develop in the student if

he insists upon discussion of pattern recognition by his teachers in clinical medicine.

PRINCIPLES IN HYPOTHESIS SETTING DERIVED FROM EXPERIENCE

The following discussion centers upon those principles enumerated initially in this chapter which serve as guidelines to the clinician. At the outset, it should be understood that such expressions of "common wisdom" are generalizations which do not always apply in a specific instance. The reader may well recognize exceptions to each guideline, which in no way detracts from their applicability or usefulness in general.

Common Diseases Occur Commonly

Among all possible causes of disease, some factors occur with great frequency and others only rarely, with a complete spectrum in between. It is obvious, but often forgotten or ignored, that the physician should always think of common causes first. Elsewhere in this text are described some of the reasons for selecting unusual, unique or rare diseases as a first thought. The rationale and application of the "commonness" concept will be considered here.

Each physician selects an area of medical practice during the course of his medical education. He concentrates his studies in that area. One consequence of this selection is that a specified population will be served. He then must learn of the status of that population in relation to health and disease. An aspiring obstetrician quickly realizes that he is dealing with a generally healthy population of women in the child-bearing years whose medical problems are few and number among them certain conditions he will encounter repetitively. Without necessarily recognizing it, he is already laying the groundwork for his hypo heses in the future.

If a woman in the age group alluded to misses two menstrual cycles, he will think most logically of pregnancy, and not of the multitude of other causes of amenorrhea, *provided there are no outstanding clues to point away from commonness.* This latter thought must underscore the discussion of common-ness. The concept applies only to those situations in which the findings can be explained both by a common cause and by uncommon ones. In these instances the physician thinks of the common causes *first*. However, if even a single element varies from the usual, the other elements are reevaluated and uncommon causes may become more likely.

"Commonness" simply is an expression of probability derived from experience. With a given set of symptoms, the largest percentage of individuals of a given sex and age group will most likely have certain diseases—not necessarily always, but most often. The frequency of each disease will determine its probability in a given set of circumstances and in a given period.

One must not be totally lulled by prior experience. Health and susceptibility to disease change constantly. Thus, a clinician cannot always be content with knowing what *was*, but he also must know what *is*. A good example of this can be found in the practice of pediatrics. Today, diseases such as measles, polio, scurvy and malnutrition are relatively rare, whereas they were major problems a few decades ago. The physician who has practiced over this span must learn to readjust his concept of commonness because the individual he encounters today with paralysis probably does not have poliovirus infection, whereas an individual 30 years ago probably would have had it. There are many such examples in medicine, and there is every reason to believe that such changes in incidence of specific diseases will continue to occur in the foreseeable future.

Although consideration of this concept can be overdone, it is important to stress certain features that physicians utilize frequently. Commonness means a high degree of probability; in statistical terms expressed as a frequency rate. Thus, the frequency of myocardial infarction in males over 50 who manifest certain characteristics of physique, life-style and habit is such that consistent symptomatology in a given member of that group must be considered evidence of infarction until proven otherwise. Actually, what is realized is that given 100 individuals of the specified population, a certain number, usually sub-stantially more than a majority, will experience that disease during the applicable time period.

If we add pattern development and recognition to the analysis, our concept of commonness can be more precisely limited. Thus, the over-50-year-old white male executive, who is more than 10 lb overweight and smokes more than 2 packages of cigarettes each day and who exercises rarely has an even higher probability of infarction than do many of his peers. In actual clinical practice the physician will come to expect that myocardial infarction is likely to occur in such an individual and may even undertake preventive measures with the patient. In this case, commonness has resulted in an hypothesis being established prior to the problem, with resulting anticipatory therapy.

In the usual clinical circumstance the physician employs the concept of commonness in sequential diagnosis. If diagnoses (hypotheses) of equal possibility are developed to explain a given set of clinical data, the physician will tend to consider the commonest one as his principal (or even only) hypothesis in subsequent problem-solving steps. If a patient presents with acute purulent tonsillopharyngitis, infection with Group A beta-hemolytic streptococci will be quickly established as the hypothesis. The physician will act as if this were the only hypothesis, and his diagnostic and therapeutic efforts will be developed in the acceptance or rejection of it.

Purulent tonsillopharyngitis can also be caused by tularemia, gonococci, tuberculosis and a variety of viral agents. Ordinarily, the clinician will not consider these possibilities because of their low probability. On the other hand, if cultures of the throat are negative for Group A streptococci, the other possibilities suddenly become more tenable and should be considered.

Unfortunately, the intellectual appeal of the exotic, the unusual, the unique or the mysterious can result in the distortion of priorities in establishing hypotheses. Too often, secondary hypotheses are prematurely elevated to primary consideration because they are intellectually attractive ideas. This temptation must be firmly resisted if the data clearly indicate more common, if mundane, explanations. This aspect of diagnosis is accentuated among practitioners who are highly specialized, and in centers accustomed to difficult diagnostic problems. In these clinical settings the expectation is one of ultimate resolution of problems. This can result in unwarranted consideration of improbable but minimally possible hypotheses. On occasion, one can encounter such exotic and unusual diagnosis raised to an equivalent level as that of the more probable commoner ones. This is the medical equivalent to the "emperor's robe" situation. In this childhood moral tale, an emperor is persuaded that he is wearing robes of the finest material and workmanship but, in fact, is wearing nothing. The persuasion comes from the belief that the wearer is unworthy if he cannot see the beauty of the invisible raiment. The folly of the emperor's vanity is unveiled by an innocent, usually a child in the variations of this tale, who exclaims, "But the Emperor is wearing no clothes!" Many of our cleverest hypotheses are like the emperor's clothes, of no substance and born of the vanity of the diagnostician.

Single Causes Explain Most Diseases

Medical practice most commonly involves acute processes. Most acute processes stem from a single cause. These are statements of probability derived from experience. Most of us are in homeostatic balance at any given point in our lives. Most frequently, disturbance in that balance occurs because a single etiologic factor is operating in our environment. Most obvious are the many and varied infectious agents which dramatically and acutely alter health by their invasion and growth. An extension of this phenomenon applies to other diseases, even if the etiology is not known. Rheumatoid arthritis, cancer, hemolytic anemia, regional enteritis and a host of varied diseases will produce a characteristic symptom-complex in an individual patient; all of the symptoms are related to the primary cause and not to multiple etiologic stimuli.

In acute disease one should therefore postulate a single cause, process or disease to account for all of the observed manifesta-

tions. For example, if a patient presents with lymphadenopathy, hepatosplenomegaly, fever, anemia, leukopenia and thrombocytopenia, it is possible that each finding has a separate explanation. Conceivably, one could establish a separate hypothesis for all six positive findings. However, it is more productive to seek a single process which explains all six findings first. Why? Because that is the statistical nature of the pathophysiology of disease. Most often a patient with an acute process manifesting these six findings will be afflicted with a single disease, not three or five or six diseases.

That some patients have multiple, simultaneously present diseases does not detract from the generalization. It does mean that the diagnostician must be able to sort out the more common diseases of single-factor causation from those less frequent multiple-causation processes.

When constructing hypotheses it is wisest to initially consider that a single process accounts for all manifestations. Only if analysis of the data in relation to such a single-cause hypothesis indicates that more than one disease is present, should this initial approach be modified.

All expressions of probability assist us in efficiency of diagnosis. At the purely abstract level, we could consider all possible explanations, mixing single and multiple causes and evaluating them simultaneously. For the majority of problems patients have, this mode of approach will be inefficient, since single causation outnumbers multiple causation by such a wide margin. For a few patients, adherence to the single-cause precept will result in delay in establishing the presence of several diseases. The facile clinician will not permit undue acceptance of *any* generalization to interfere with the solution of his patient's individual problem. Although the probability of a patient having systemic lupus erythematosus and rheumatoid arthritis simultaneously is remote, for the patient who is so afflicted the possibility is 100%.

Simple Problems Should Lead to Simple Hypotheses

If a patient complains of a sore throat and has an inflamed pharynx, one chooses the simplest explanation, e.g., an infection. It is *possible* that the sore throat is due to a complex cerebral process which causes that abnormal sensation, but it is *probable* that the simpler explanation is correct.

In our highly complex medical practice the temptation to evoke complex explanations for seemingly straightforward phenomenon is always present. It is intellectually satisfying to both know and express the rare, the complex, the intricate and the fascinating. For all the satisfaction such intellectual meanderings have, they have little place in most diagnostic practice. Most diseases are extensions of simple pathophysiologic processes.

Even those that appear complex can have a simple explanation. Consider the 55-year-old female patient with vaginal moniliasis, early cataracts, obesity, peripheral vascular insufficiency in the distal extremities and atherosclerotic cardiovascular disease with congestive heart failure. This combination of findings is related to the presence of diabetes mellitus or, more simply, to lack of insulin effect. This example illustrates the concept of "simple" causation. By *simple* is not meant trivial or unimportant or unworthy of attention. Rather, *simple* refers to the uncomplicated, straightforward, noncomplex explanation.

Hypotheses Should Be Derived from the Data, Not in Reverse Order

The physician must constantly remember that his explanations for a given pattern of findings in a patient are based upon those findings. This seems so self-evident as not to require statement. However, one common diagnostic misapplication is to become fixed upon a disease entity and attempt to fit the patient's findings into it. For example, one student learned, early in his career, a great deal about lupus erythematosus. He was knowledgeable concerning this disease out of proportion to his general medical store of information. Upon reaching the clinical instruction period he tended to label most patients with difficult diagnostic problems as lupus. In each instance he molded the patient's history and physical findings to conform to lupus in all of its variations. He almost never was correct. Only with increased

clinical experience and the amassing of considerable factual knowledge did he temper his diagnostic enthusiasm for lupus erythematosus.

Such an extreme example may seem aberrant and fail to reflect the bulk of medical practice. However, many instances of this phenomenon occur daily in medicine. Common examples include (1) believing that vitamin deficiency is a cause for a variety of patient complaints; (2) diagnosing hypothyroidism for any complaint involving fatigue, lassitude, loss of ambition, etc.; (3) diagnosing immunodeficiency in patients who have recurrent respiratory infections, to the point of prescribing monthly gamma-globulin therapy; and (4) attempting to establish an organic explanation for most psychologic and behavioral disorders. There are many other examples. All have several common features: The diagnosis is usually in the mind of the clinician prior to collection of any, or all, of the data; the diagnosis is decided prior to, or in spite of, contradictory laboratory data; and usually there is a treatment attached to the erroneous label.

The basic positive assumption should be that the patient's manifestations are indicative of some pathophysiologic process. A good diagnostician approaches each problem as a fresh one. Each patient is his own source of stimuli to the problem-solving process. Each individual reacts to the causes of disease and expresses those processes. Therefore, the clinician looks to the patient and not the textbook for his primary hypotheses.

The Utilization of Pathophysiology in Establishing Hypotheses

One very successful approach to diagnosis is the interpretation of all data in the light of known pathophysiologic processes. One can treat jaundice as a symptom in a variety of ways: as an expression of hyperbilirubinemia, as an excretory product of the liver, as a breakdown product of hemoglobin or as an element in a complex metabolic cycle which can go awry.

The latter approach, that of the pathophysiologic process, is usually the most productive avenue of analysis. To the extent that we can explain normal physiologic mechanisms and their tissue and organ relationships, we can understand the production of symptoms, the appearance of physical changes in the body, and the causes of deviations detectable in the laboratory. For some systems, the cerebral and peripheral nervous systems, for example, this approach is not yet practically feasible or, at best, is only a superficial attempt made for some processes. But for most systems and diseases, a modest to extensive mapping of pathophysiology is known, even though etiology may be unknown.

Analysis by pathophysiologic processes can permit anticipation of the course of disease and also be used to judge therapy. In testing an hypothesis founded in pathophysiology, validity can be determined more readily if a predictable outcome is anticipated. For example, if excessive destruction of erythrocytes is postulated in an instance of anemia and jaundice, the administration of Cr*-labeled erythrocytes and the observation of their fate can establish the validity of the destruction hypothesis. One can also predict deposition of bilirubin in various tissues and, by observing it, verify the premise. If the destruction is postulated to be due to an antibody interacting with the erythrocyte, therapy designed to suppress this antibody or minimize the effects of its interaction can be selected, and the response evaluated.

Many examples in clinical practice illustrate the value of the pathophysiologic approach. In some clinical circumstances the diagnostician may not know the disease present in his patient but nonetheless arrive at a sound understanding of its effects by analyzing the aberrant physiology. Frequently one can arrive at a diagnosis of an infectious or inflammatory process without being able, at that moment, to identify the specific cause.

Knowledge and application of pathophysiologic principles enables us to sort and weigh clinical data. Symptoms which do not fit an otherwise sound pathophysiologic explanation may be (1) inaccurate patient perceptions, (2) symptomatic of a coexisting process, including psychologic ones, or (3) indicative of an error in the reasoning. Once again, the clinician must be wary, lest facts are made to fit his concept of pathophysiology rather than the reverse.

Interpretation of initial data on pathophysiologic grounds can lead to fruitful additional search for data. In a jaundiced patient whose problem appears to stem from impaired excretion of bilirubin, a search for subtle signs of liver or biliary disease not originally uncovered may be indicated. In the patient with bacterial sepsis following heart valve damage, one would look for cerebral and renal involvement, knowing the pathophysiologic sequences inherent in this disease pattern.

Pathophysiologic hypotheses are usually stated in mechanistic terms rather than as disease states or specific syndromes. One's vista is then less clouded by the obscurity of "somebody's syndrome" and is facilitated by the sequential process implicit in the nomenclature. A patient who expresses signs and symptoms of combined immunodeficiency with antibody and cell-mediated immune deficit has a more clearly defined pathophysiologic process than is implied by the label "Swiss-type hypogammaglobulinemia." The label given a disease state does not change the manifestations of that disease in any way. The pathophysiologically oriented descriptors simply facilitate appreciation of the underlying processes and more clearly express what is going on. In the nomenclature of hypotheses, it permits accurate statement which can make testing of the hypotheses more systematic. However, the label alone will not improve the diagnostician's effort.

The Use of Multiple Hypotheses

All diagnosticians strive for the single best hypothesis that explains all of the facts. In actual practice this striving is frequently successful. But not always. For this reason, one should be prepared to make multiple suggestions to explain some sets of data. This is especially true in the instance of few available data of nonspecific nature; in these instances many causes of approximately equal probability can account for the findings. The following case is an example of this clinical phenomenon:

A newborn infant was delivered to a nulliparous woman following an uncomplicated pregnancy, labor and delivery. The male child was full-term, weighing 6 lb 12 oz, and appeared normal grossly at birth. The child became anorexic and listless within 48 hours and was discovered to have an enlarged liver (2 cm below the right costal margin in the nipple line) and spleen (1 cm below the left costal margin in the anterior axillary line). No other symptoms or signs were evident.

This child did not display sufficiently specific signs or symptoms that permitted a quickly established single hypothesis. Many infectious, hematologic, metabolic and cerebral causes could be invoked to explain the findings. Only by a multiple-hypotheses approach could the search be conducted logically. At the outset, each possibility was of equal probability, given the paucity and nonspecificity of the findings; only following a wide search was the field narrowed to infectious etiology and from there to congenital cytomegalovirus infection. Since the probability of finding any of the several possibilities was equal or near-equal, the clinician could not confine himself to a sequential search but needed to probe in several areas simultaneously.

Another useful area for multiple hypotheses is the disease or condition which is life-threatening and may have a treatable cause. In such instances, one must consider more than one explanation in order not to miss a correctable deficit. The comatose patient, the child in shock, the infant with renal failure, the patient with signs of meningitis—all present a mandate for complete diagnostic evaluation. Among the causes for each are included those for which specific therapy may be life-saving. To consider only diabetic coma in a comatose child is to condemn some children with head trauma and intracranial bleeding to sure demise, when neurosurgical intervention may be life-saving.

To the initiate it is often confusing to find a teacher emphasizing both the single-best-hypothesis and the multiple-hypotheses approaches. This is the nature of the problems encountered in clinical medicine. As will be emphasized later, no single diagnostic method will do for all problems. The clinician must be facile, using one approach for this specific problem and another for a differing problem. What is being attempted in this chapter is to demonstrate the many ways of establishing hypotheses with some insight into when to employ a specific approach.

The Flexibility of Setting and Retaining Hypotheses

At no point should the student develop the idea that the problem-solving process is a fixed, rigid structure. One of the difficulties computer scientists have had in attempting to simulate human problem solving completely is the tremendous flexibility inherent in the process.

As the clinician is introduced to the patient and his problem(s), he instantly begins the process of problem solving. With the very first data collection, he begins making testable assumptions. In fact, he may do so *before* actually meeting the patient in person. The initial contact may be a phone call, or an entry in his appointment book, or a conversation with another physician. Immediately, he begins learning some facts about the patient, and the process is underway. Such factors as age, sex and social and economic status may serve to establish preliminary background for the first complaint or symptom. From that point on, if the physician is more than a data collector, he will establish, discard, modify, expand, contract and otherwise alter hypotheses. Problem solving is an extremely fluid and dynamic process, and attempts to chart it always fall short because all of the arrows and feedback circuits cannot be indicated. At most, we can surmise the general flow from data through hypothesis, through testing to conclusion and action and/or inaction. During any actual exercise of problem solving the process flows rapidly back and forth between these stopping points and may be blurred beyond recognition.

Even the simplest problems and hypotheses have such a pattern, even though it is implemented with lightning speed, and at a level of consciousness almost beyond recall. In complex problems it is easier to see this seesawing of reasoning and judgement. Perusal of any clinicopathologic discussion reveals to some extent the mental gymnastics of the diagnostician.

Therefore, in approaching problem solving, an initiate should not hesitate to make assumptions based on initial data, testing their validity as the interview and examination progresses. One must be prepared to alter or discard any of them as new facts emerge. A conclusion should be formed, provided one always recognizes its inherent instability and is willing to quickly adjust, given more information.

A student can directly benefit from his teacher's experience and wisdom. The teacher must be persuaded to expose the early stages of reasoning to the student. He should be able to show the student how and why they went from A → B → C → D → E. They should describe the reasons for rejected early hypotheses and for later reconsideration. Whatever the particular process was should be made evident. It is a student's responsibility to study and command the problem-solving process. A good way to understand it more fully is to dissect, or have dissected, the reasoning of more experienced performers, i.e., the teacher of medicine.

Similarly, when reading a case discussion, a journal article dealing with disease analysis, or a clinicopathologic conference, the student should look for this process and its ramifications. Consciously drawn inferences should be made by the reader and compared with those of the discussants. This exercise will prove of great value if diligently pursued. It is an excellent self-discipline which can improve problem-solving skills.

Medical Logic

Underlying all hypothesis setting is a sense of medical logic. Logical thinking in medicine does not differ from that observed in other intellectual endeavors.

Logic can be defined simply as the science and art of clear thinking. It is the science of symbolic or abstract thought. By clear thinking is meant many things, including the recognition, appreciation and manipulation of the attributes and relationships of ideas. By medical logic we ordinarily mean the individual's ability to think clearly about the relationships between individual bits of medical information; that is, to be able to perceive facts concerning human normality and abnormality and to apply these facts to prob-

lems involving their relationships in an orderly fashion.

Medical thought is filled with examples of logical reasoning. Basically there are two types: inductive and deductive reasoning.

By *inductive reasoning* is meant the ability to generalize from the particular. If observations are made about the character, attributes or function of individual objects, inductive reasoning permits us to formulate propositions that are universally true for all individual things of the type observed. For example, we might observe that individual automobiles each have a steering wheel; we may then generalize, formulating the hypothesis (or theory or proposition) that all automobiles have steering wheels. Certain factors will make this proposition a "good" one to arrive at, or a poor one. Is the sample of observation large enough to permit the establishment of an hypothesis? Have the individual bits of data been collected randomly? Or is there present the bias of some selective process? How accurate are the observations? How much variability is there in the observer? In the object being observed?

An inductively reasoned hypothesis will stand or fall, partially on the basis of these additional factors. Also, a further dimension of validity is the extent to which the hypothesis can be tested and either accepted or rejected. This topic will be dealt with in Chapter 5.

Induction is used by research workers in medicine, by medical theorists and philosophers and by clinicians. The clinician utilizes inductive reasoning in the establishment of clinical hypotheses based upon his observations, the patient's verbal reports, and the results of laboratory data.

Deductive reasoning is the process of moving from the universal or general "truth" to the particular or specific instance. Thus, the sequence, (*1*) all men must die, (*2*) John is a man, (*3*) therefore, John must die, is a deductive one. Deductions are as valid as the general assumption is true and provided the specific instance is a correct example of the generalization. To assert from Step *1* above that a specific *dog* must die cannot be deduced from the general truth about *men*.

Deduction is used frequently in the diagnostic process, usually after an hypothesis has been set. The clinician uses the sequence: (*1*) Disease X has certain characteristics; (*2*) the patient has 80% of these characteristics; (*3*) therefore, the patient has the disease.

It is obvious from this example that the clinician makes a statistical deduction rather than an absolute one. The difficulty with most medical deductions is the unavailability of many universal "truths" and the nature of the "specific" data, which often makes them less specific than pure logical sequence demands. Nevertheless, physicians use deduction frequently, even if only in a statistical (or probability) sense. In the medical example given above, the correct deduction is (*3*)—it is highly probably that this patient has disease X.

The physician must be wary of all of the logical fallacies. As used here, the logical fallacy is the sequential thought pattern that *appears* logical but, on closer scrutiny, is not. The usual types of logical fallacy encountered in medicine can be subdivided as follows: (1) intended fallacies or sophisms, (2) fallacies of expression or language, (3) fallacies of "accident," (4) fallacy of the qualified versus the absolute statement, (5) fallacy of irrelevant conclusions, (6) fallacy of begging the question, (7) fallacy of false cause, (8) fallacy of the consequent proving the antecedent, (9) fallacy of many questions, (10) fallacy of *non sequitur*, (11) fallacy of appeal to ignorance, (12) fallacy of suppressing the facts, (13) fallacy of argument from silence, (14) fallacy of false assumption, (15) fallacy of illicit generalization and (16) fallacy of false analogy. A brief consideration of each of these fallacies is important to both our consideration of the establishment of hypotheses and general medical thought.

Sophisms are frequently encountered in medical advertising. They can take the form of any of the specific types of fallacy. For the diagnostic process the significance of sophism lies in the use of this device to establish an hypothesis which supports the clinician's bias rather than stems from the data. Obviously, intended fallacies are to be avoided by the physician with integrity.

Fallacies of expression or language are varied. Aristotle originally listed six major categories: equivocation, amphiboly, composition, division, accent and figures of speech.

Equivocation occurs when a word is used in a sense different from its meaning. In pure logical argument the following sequence is an example: (*1*) What is natural is good; (*2*) but to make mistakes is natural; (*3*) therefore, to make mistakes is good. The equivocation here is in the use of the varied-meaning word *natural*; it means one thing in (*1*) and quite a different thing in (*2*). A medical example is as follows: (*1*) One characteristic of rheumatoid arthritis is arthritis; (*2*) this patient has arthritis; (*3*) therefore, this patient has rheumatoid arthritis. The term "arthritis" has a definition as used in (*1*). If in (*2*), however, the patient actually has arthralgia or neuritis or myalgia, the deduction is fallacious.

Amphiboly is the use of an ambiguous phrase in a logical argument. This is actually just an extension of equivocation.

Composition refers to the use of a group of thoughts as one and then excepting any member from the universality attributed to the group. In formal logic an example would be: (*1*) Lying and cheating are deplorable; (*2*) I am only a liar, not a cheat; (*3*) therefore, I am not deplorable. The fallacy lies in considering lying and cheating as a unit rather than as separate qualities, either of which is deplorable. In medicine: (*1*) Pneumonia is characterized by cough, fever and productive sputum; (*2*) this patient has only cough and fever; (*3*) therefore, this patient does not have pneumonia. The error of composition should be obvious.

Divisional fallacies are the opposite of compositional ones. That is, members of an inseparable group are taken individually. From formal logic: (*1*) All in this room weigh 2 tons; (*2*) Mary is in this room; (*3*) therefore, Mary weighs 2 tons. From medicine: (*1*) Fever, rash and coryza are characteristic of measles; (*2*) this patient has fever; (*3*) therefore, this patient has measles.

Fallacies of accent refer to the emphasis placed upon one of a collection of attributes. In formal logic: (*1*) A person should not tell lies about his neighbors' faults. By emphasizing "lies," it is implied that it is alright to tell truths about the neighbors' faults. By emphasizing "neighbor," it is implied that lies can be told about nonneighbors' behavior, and so forth. In medicine: (*1*) Antibiotics should not be given to patients with unsubstantiated infectious diseases. One can conclude that it is proper to give antibiotics to patients with substantiated infectious diseases or even to administer them to patients with noninfectious diseases, depending upon the emphasis or "accent" given.

The fallacy involving *figures of speech* is, strictly speaking, a play on words and has less significance for medical practice than for medical advertising.

The *fallacy of accident* is the use of an incidental quality of a particular thing to establish its true nature. In classical logic: (*1*) You say you ate what you bought; (*2*) but you bought raw meat; (*3*) therefore, you ate raw meat? The confusion here stems from the selection of the "rawness" of the meat from among its qualities, which also includes edibility upon cooking, which was not selected. In medicine: This patient is 30-years-old and has a lump in her breast and a family history of cancer and has noticed like lumps during each menstrual cycle and is having a period at present. To argue that the lumps must be cancerous *because* of her positive family history would be an example of the fallacy of accident.

The *confusion of absolute and qualified statements* is common in medicine. Two kinds of fallacious reasoning are included: the use of a restricted truth in a universal sense, and the assumption of implied generalization when, in fact, no such generalization exists in the principle quoted. An example of the first type from formal logic: (*1*) Italians can be excellent opera singers; (*2*) therefore, this Italian is an excellent opera singer. In medicine: (*1*) Patients with penicillin antibodies can have anaphylactic reactions to penicillin; (*2*) therefore, this patient with penicillin antibodies will have an anaphylactic reaction to penicillin. What is lacking are all of the conditions under which (*1*) is true and a comparison of those conditions with the state of the particular patient.

An example of the second type from formal logic is: (*1*) He gave me $1,000 of counterfeit money; (*2*) therefore, he gave me $1,000. The statement in (*2*) is *not* implied by (*1*). From medicine: (*1*) This patient has some of the symptoms of subacute bacterial endocarditis; (*2*) therefore, it can be anticipated that this patient will manifest all of the symptoms of subacute bacterial endocarditis. The former is restricted; the latter, too generalized and *not* implied in the former.

The use of *irrelevant conclusions* is one of the more common fallacies; it is appealing because the conclusion seems logical. For example, a trial lawyer inveighs against the injustice done to his client without paying any attention to the evidence that the defendant is guilty or innocent. Although seemingly logical, and obviously not, this type of fallacy pervades everyday thinking: "He is such a nice guy, he couldn't have embezzled all that money," "he doesn't look like a doctor" (or lawyer or congressman or almost anything!) "I don't trust her, did you see the way she wears her hair?" and so forth.

In medicine this fallacy is encountered often in the judgements made about a patient's illness that are based upon an irrelevant characteristic or characteristics. Utilizing some personal feature—race, sex, social status, economic position, appearance, cleanliness (or lack of it), ethnic origin, etc.—the physician makes an *unwarranted* judgement concerning illness. A clear distinction must be made between statistically associated diseases and the above traits, which is legitimate, and the irrelevant associations, which are not. To consider all housewives as "flighty" and diagnose anxiety neurosis on the basis of this irrelevancy is one example. Others include assuming all poor people (or blacks or Puerto Ricans or Eskimos) have "worms," all rising young executives have ulcers, all teenagers are drug addicts, etc. Nor are all errors of fallacy made in a negative sense. Some physicians conclude that because this patient is a well-educated professional, he automatically understands medical terminology. Or that an adolescent from a "good" home cannot have venereal disease or be pregnant. The physician is so familiar with relevant comparisons between personal characteristics and disease states that sometimes it is difficult to avoid irrelevant conclusions.

Begging the question is also a commonly encountered fallacy in everyday life as well as in medical practice. This fallacy takes several forms but, in general, involves using a conclusion (rightly or wrongly assumed) to prove a component of that conclusion. Thus: (*1*) Federal government programs are bad;

(2) this is a Federal program; (3) therefore, this is a bad program. Or, (1) All patients with ulcers are neurotic; (2) this patient has an ulcer; (3) therefore, this patient is neurotic.

Another form of begging the question is to state the conclusion in different terms but with the same meaning as the assertion. Thus: "The soul is immortal *because* it cannot die." In medicine: Cortisone is the best treatment for rheumatoid arthritis because cortisone is anti-inflammatory.

Yet other forms include circular reasoning and the use of prejudicial language.

The *fallacy of false cause* finds its presence in many therapeutic claims in medicine based upon temporal association. In formal logic, false cause arises from infusing a causal relationship with a noncausal one. This is the *"post hoc, ergo propter hoc"* fallacy (after this, therefore, because of this). "Winter follows summer; therefore, summer causes winter." Absurd? Of course, but consider, "The patient got well after I gave him penicillin; therefore, he got well because I gave him penicillin." Or, "patients with the common cold whom I treat with chloramphenicol all get well! Therefore, chloramphenicol is indicated in the common cold." Examples of this type of fallacy abound in medicine. Anecdotal evidence of a cause and effect relationship between a therapeutic maneuver and a desired clinical effect is frequent. Seemingly intelligent individuals are willing to accept fallacies of false cause simply because of a temporal association between events.

The *consequent fallacy* consists of establishing the truth or falsity of an antecedent because its consequent is true or false. From classical logic: (1) A dog is an animal; (2) a cat is an animal; (3) therefore, a cat is a dog. In a negative sense the same facts can lead to: (1) A dog is an animal; (2) a cat is not a dog; (3) therefore, a cat is not an animal. From medicine: (1) Antibiotics cure infection by destroying bacteria; (2) colds may be due to bacteria; (3) therefore, antibiotics can cure colds.

The *fallacy of many questions* results from seeking simple answers to complex or multiple-component questions. For example, a favorite courtroom technique is to ask for a yes-or-no answer to a multiple-component question, such as "Is the defendant a man who is easily aroused to anger and capable of fatally injuring another person?" It can be clearly seen that a simple yes or no answer cannot be given if the defendant is easily aroused to anger but incapable of inflicting fatal injuries. By tying two seemingly related questions together and demanding a simple answer, one appears to link the two characteristics. In medicine this fallacy is expressed usually by linking together processes or characteristics in a given patient and testing for one and assuming the result substantiates both. This topic will be dealt with in greater detail in Chapter 5.

Non-sequitur arguments are fallacious because the conclusion does not follow from the premises. A classic example, which is obviously absurd, is: (1) Cows give milk; (2) but sheep have wool; (3) therefore, goats chew cud. Trivial examples are plentiful, and the obviousness of the fallacy usually prevents major errors. In medicine this fallacy is occasionally encountered in situations similar to the following: (1) This patient has a severe case of pancreatitis; (2) carcinoma of the pancreas frequently causes obstruction of the bile duct leading to jaundice; (3) therefore, this patient's jaundice must be due to obstruction of the common bile duct. The subtle juxtaposition of the pathophysiologic concomitant of one disease (carcinoma of the pancreas) to the symptom of another (pancreatitis) affecting the same organ seems (superficially) to make sense but does not withstand scrutiny.

Appeal to ignorance implies truth because a premise cannot be refuted; and it implies falsity because of lack of proof. Hence, this patient has myocarditis because it cannot be proven he doesn't! Farfetched? Unfortunately not, there are many examples of therapeutic justification based upon the fallacy of appeal to ignorance.

Suppressing the facts is one of the commonest fallacies encountered in the establishment of hypotheses by selection of facts that fit and by suppression, conscious or not, of those bits of data which do not conform. This fallacy has been adequately discussed elsewhere in this chapter.

Arguing from silence has little applicability in medicine. It consists of arguing that something asserted would have been recorded if it were true; therefore, it must be false in the absence of documentation. A variant is occasionally encountered in medicine in such statements as: "If this drug were dangerous, they never would have developed or licensed it."

A *false assumption* is actually an error. This fallacy has been adequately explored throughout this book. Assumption of a fact or premise which is not true obviously renders subsequent reasoning incorrect.

Illicit generalization consists of making a generalization on insufficient data. Again, this fallacy has been covered throughout this chapter and will not be further detailed here.

False analogy refers to inaccurate use of similarities between two things to infer characteristics of one from characteristics of the other. Argument by analogy is a legitimate tool of reasoning and logic. False analogy is fallacious because its conclusions rest upon similarities that are unrelated to the trait or characteristic under consideration. For example, individuals A and B may be of similar weight, height and muscle mass. Arguing by analogy, one can assert similar physical strength. A false analogy would be the assertion of similar intelligence, since intelligence is not related to physique.

This digression into logic and the common fallacies is included because the establishment of hypotheses requires logical thought and the avoidance of fallacy. Hypotheses are born of inductive or deductive thought processes following principles of logic.

Clinicians differ in their approach to problem solving as discussed in Chapter 2. Such differences are referred to as "style" and reflect individual variation in the logical approach to problem solving. This phenomenon is possible because there is no absolute, unbending methodology to clinical diagnosis. Rather, a series of alternative methods are utilized in reaching reasonable conclusions from the same data.

The alternatives are as varied as the clinicians employing them, or so it seems. Actually, there are relatively few "styles" into which most variations fit. These have been discussed in Chapter 2. The pertinence of this phenomenon for the topic under discussion is revealed in an analysis of the styles of problem solving. Central to most variations

and implicit in the alternatives are the varied methods by which hypotheses are established.

Thus, one broad group of clinicians will use an "intuitive" or "hunch" approach depending upon unseen forces within themselves for selecting the correct choice(s) from among all of those data stored subconsciously. Unkind critics refer to this method as an unconscious or mindless approach. In actual practice it tends to replace thinking with "inspiration." A variety of motivations and other factors are inherent in this method. Laziness, fatigue, a facile mind, impatience, lack of knowledge, mystical belief in one's powers—all can be concealed beneath the employment of this technique by individual physicians. In fact, most clinicians will lapse into an haphazard approach given the appropriate circumstances, e.g., fatigue, necessity for haste occasioned by too many commitments, etc. Only the most disciplined escape occasional or rare lapses into intuitive diagnosis. Whether employed by someone else or employed personally, the student can discover this methodology if the answer to the "why" of hypothesis selection is "I don't know." For every other alternative, reasons, correct or incorrect, can be offered for the choice of hypotheses. From the preceding discussion it must be obvious to the student that this method is lightly regarded. It is the province of amateurs and dilettantes, and its consistent use is to be deplored. On occasion, intuitive diagnosis is the result of undefinable associations based upon the data, in which the "correct" answer is "obvious," even without the diagnostician's ability to trace his reasoning, step by step.

A second broad category of hypothesis setting is that of the differential diagnosis. In this instance the clinician weighs each bit of data, attempts to discern a pattern or patterns among them and then fits them into the known causes of that pattern or patterns. In its most compulsive form this process results in the establishment of a list of all possibilities, a list which is limited only by the scope of the diagnostician's knowledge and by his ability to discriminate patterns of data accurately.

The art and science of differential diagnosis have been the subject of many scientific papers, lectures and textbooks. Common to all of these is the attempt to weigh the data in reference to its "match" or "fit" with the known characteristics of a given disease, state or condition. Some authors advise selecting a single symptom, sign or laboratory finding that is the most specific available. The ultimate expression of specificity is found in the pathognomonic sign. If the observer detects Koplik's spot on the buccal mucosa of an individual, he can leap to the diagnosis of measles without fear of error. Unfortunately, few findings are that specific. Given an individual with weakness (subjective), anorexia and bloody diarrhea, one would focus upon bloody diarrhea, as it is the most specific of the data. If the patient presents with cyanosis, a characteristic murmur, measured hepatomegaly, and moist rales, one is confronted with multiple specific signs whose pattern may be specific enough to focus upon in establishing the list of hypotheses. Thus, one method for proceeding from data to hypothesis is based upon selection of specific data of high specificity and drawing your conclusions from that particular vantage point.

Other authors recommend the use of "symptom-complexes" or those combinations of findings that suggest diagnoses. In reality this is an extension of the specific clue method, but not completely. A combination of nonspecific cues may constitute a specific pattern or cluster. Thus, malaise, fever, cough, weight loss and anorexia taken together may carry more "weight" in the diagnosis of certain chronic diseases (tuberculosis, pyelonephritis, malignancy) than do any of the separate findings. Cluster analysis requires a high degree of ability to relate isolated bits of data, giving more or less weight to members included in, and excluded from, the cluster. In a patient with multiple subjective symptoms and findings on examination, one must be able to discern accurately the relatedness of certain members of the total array and, also, to recognize major and minor contributors to the process. This form of diagnosis reaches its peak in the clinical formulae utilized to recognize rheumatic fever or rheumatoid arthritis. In fact, most of the so-called collagen vascular diseases have such varied and nonspecific manifestations that

only by a combinational approach can diagnosis be achieved.

Yet other clinicians suggest that each and all findings be used to determine a differential diagnosis. In this method an elaborate grid work (written or mental) is constructed with the diagnosis consistent with each finding ranging along one axis and each finding along the other. In this way, compatible diagnoses are matched with the entire range of findings. Some computer programs for diagnosis have utilized a similar approach to differential diagnosis. One limitation of this method is the necessary assignment of weight to the data. There is little allowance for such vagaries of data as "possible splenomegaly." A strict match between findings and diagnosis is basically dependent upon the findings, their precision, relative value in analysis of the illness, and relative meaning in the pathophysiologic process. The best differential diagnostic approaches are found in those clinical instances which yield "hard" data. Examples include fluid and electrolyte disturbances, renal dysfunction or failure, various respiratory disorders and some lesions of the central nervous system. So-called geographic diseases, in the sense of anatomic location, also lend themselves readily to this approach. Masses in the various portions of the mediastinum, cerebral space-occupying lesions, abdominal masses, forms of intestinal obstruction, and many other anatomically confined processes can be successfully analyzed as to nature, by application of the finding-differential diagnosis grid-work. Also, diseases with clearly defined and almost universal manifestations can be processed in this fashion; metabolic defects, immunologic deficiencies, chromosomal syndromes and congenital cardiovascular diseases—all fit this pattern.

The vaguer the symptoms and signs, and the less we know of the pathophysiology of the disease, the more difficult it is to utilize the mathematical precision of differential diagnosis.

All modes of diagnosis or hypothesis formulation can be fit within the framework of these broad categories. Almost all observed or described methods are variations on one of these themes. The facility with which any method is utilized is very dependent upon the physician's powers of concentration, his intelligence, his memory and his unique ability to handle multiple variables in complex relationships. This skill is partially dependent upon innate talents, but a good deal of it can be acquired. The student should polish the necessary talents by endless practice, by continuous exercise of his mind. No problem is too small, too trivial or too mundane to allow the physician to bypass the process. Thinking is what the entire practice of medicine is all about.

One other aspect of the establishment of hypotheses deserves mention. No diagnostician *always* uses the same method for every problem. A given approach may be utilized much more frequently than another, but the variety of problems that are presented necessitates considerable flexibility. A strict differential diagnosis grid work may evolve for one problem, and a more directive single-hypothesis approach be applied to a second. The most talented diagnosticians usually are the most facile. They permit the problem and its data to lead to the system they will use and not the reverse. What works well for mediastinal masses may not do for diarrhea, or arthritis, or low-back pain. The ease with which the physician slips from one mode of establishing hypotheses to another is usually coincidental with his overall diagnostic abilities. Fixed, rigid use of a single approach is bound to result in inefficiency in some situations and outright damage to the patient in a few.

SUMMARY AND EXTENDED COMMENTS

This section has dealt with the establishment of hypotheses. Hypotheses in clinical medicine are potential explanations formulated to account for a specific patient's signs, symptoms and laboratory findings. They may be simple or complex, single or multiple, or of high probability or low probability. Regardless of their character they are formulated because they permit subsequent stages in problem solving. A well-stated hypothesis allows testing of its validity by either diagnostic or therapeutic maneuvers or both. Hypotheses may be accepted or rejected as a result of their further steps.

Some general principles, based upon cumulative medical experience, can assist the physician in formulating hypotheses. These principles are enumerated and discussed. They serve only as broad guidelines to function in many repeatedly experienced clinical problems.

Throughout this section the frame of reference has been the physician as solver of problems. In actual medical practice, currently and in the foreseeable future, other health personnel and certain mechanical systems have, and will, assume a portion of this function.

Physician's assistants are capable of problem-solving activity if their education has incorporated experience in this area *and* if their practice situation is permissive. The original conception of a physician's assistant as a collector of data whose primary function was to extend the physician's time has been altered as this health position has developed. Many trainees in this area today complete curricula designed to expose them to problem solving in the clinic or hospital. Together with the intelligence and preparation of the individual, such exposure allows experiential development of problem-solving ability.

In practice situations, physician's assistants can, and do, solve clinical problems daily. In so doing they should employ exactly the same process discussed in this book. The physician's role, for those patients and those problems encountered by the physician's assistant, is that of monitor. In order to gauge the effectiveness and accuracy of decision making by an associated physician's assistant, the physician must have a command of the problem-solving process.

Ever since the development of computer science, many have expressed the belief that the medical diagnostic process could be automated. The most extreme enthusiasts believed that it would be simple to establish a computer program which given the raw clinical data would quickly select the correct, or most appropriate, hypotheses. Realism has dictated a more modest accomplishment. A number of clinical situations have yielded to computer technology. For example, chromosomal defects have been successfully "programed," such that if the computer is given enough specific data, a specific syndrome can be offered with a high degree of probability. The instances which adapt best to computer programing are those in which clear distinction can be made between diagnoses. Also important is the relative stability of the signs, symptoms and findings in a given condition. Thus, in chromosomal defects many of the syndromes are unique and contain sufficiently distinct and constant findings to permit computer discrimination. On the other hand, many of the diseases we deal with in medicine are more variable in expression and more difficult to distinguish from similar conditions. To date, the computer fares less well with this type of discrimination.

An offshoot of computer mathematics is the development of the clinical algorithm. This is a system of choices, usually *yes* or *no*, in response to a question as to the presence or absence of a symptom, sign or laboratory finding. As the diagnostician supplies information gained from his patient, he moves along a so-called decision tree. The exact path he follows is dictated by the clinical data. If the data is sufficiently distinct *and* the condition is diagnosable given distinct data, the path will lead to a correct diagnosis. An example may help to clarify the process:

10-year-old girl with acute history of fever
Localized symptoms?

yes   no

Back pain?

yes   no

Dysuria?

yes   no

WBC and bacteria in urine?

yes   no

Acute pyelonephritis

This is a greatly simplified algorithm, but the principles are clearly illustrated. The questions at the decision point should be crisp and an answerable *yes* or *no*. *Maybe*, or any other vague answer, invalidates the usual progression in an algorithm. The conclusion must be one of *very high probability*, given the appropriate answers in the chain preceding its selection. The higher the probability, the greater the value of the algorithm.

For the foreseeable future, individual problem solving by physicians or their delegates or surrogates will continue to be a central phenomenon in medical practice. The ability to set appropriate hypotheses at the proper point in the data collection process will remain a critical element.

Chapter 5

The Testing of Hypotheses

INTRODUCTION

A well-formulated hypothesis derived from judicious weighing of historical and physical examination data is not an end unto itself. Hypotheses are developed to be working explanations for the patient's problem(s). They permit the physician to test for probable cause of the problem(s). They are frameworks upon which additional data can be placed. And finally, a soundly derived hypothesis(es) guides the physician to specific investigation rather than to haphazard search.

In testing clinical hypothesis several general guidelines direct the clinician. Among these are:

1. *An indirect approach* to accepting or rejecting a hypothesis may be the only available recourse.
2. The clinician attempts to *sample* morphology or physiologic and psychologic function.
3. Testing should be *specific and directed* to answer a question rather than be random or independent of the hypothesis.
4. The more *specific* the hypothesis, the more *precise* the testing.

These guidelines will be considered in greater detail in this chapter. An examination of the usual categories of hypothesis testing will be discussed, including (1) regularly available laboratory procedures, (2) special laboratory procedures, (3) regularly available roentgenologic examinations, (4) special roentgenologic procedures, (5) additional historical information, (6) additional physical examination data, (7) surgical procedures, (8) therapeutic trials, and (9) observation as a "test."

THE NATURE OF TESTING: INDIRECT TESTING OF HYPOTHESIS

It would be convenient if all clinical hypotheses could be tested for validity directly. That is, if a clinician believes process X is effecting tissue Y, a direct measure of the process in that tissue would ensue. Unfortunately, for the bulk of medical practice, direct testing is either impossible or not technically feasible.

Limitations in obtaining a direct test result from the hazards of performance in the patient. For example, the usual patient with mild pneumonia is not a subject for lung biopsy, even though the latter procedure is the most "direct" test for the hypothesis.

An additional limitation is encountered in those processes for which a direct assessment is not available. For example, infectious hepatitis in many instances can only be tested for indirectly, there being no direct test available.

In those situations in which direct clinical testing is either prohibited or unavailable, the diagnostician resorts to indirect measurement. Some examples may help to characterize the necessity for, and certain features of, indirect testing:

A 19-year-old male has abdominal pain, mucosanguineous diarrhea and a barely distinguishable mass in the right midabdomen. Differential diagnosis includes, among other possibilities, regional enteritis and infectious colitis. One theoretical, direct approach would be immediate laparotomy. There is little question that a specific answer probably could be obtained, especially if the process was regional enteritis. However, to do so would incur a risk for the patient; the formation of intra-abdominal fistulae commonly follows laparotomy in this condition. The most direct test, therefore, cannot be applied in this instance despite its theoretical advantage.

A 15-year-old boy presents with headache, loss of lateral motion of his eyes (paralysis of conjugate gaze), hyperreflexia of the deep tendon reflexes on the right side, truncal ataxia and horizontal nystagmus. This is sufficient data to strongly suspect a tumor, or other space-occupying lesion, in the brainstem. The most direct approach would be to view and biopsy, or remove, the tumor. Technically, this is not feasible, and such a direct answer is not available to the clinician. In instances of this type the direct approach cannot be undertaken because of technical impossibility or intrinsic lethal risk.

In both examples a direct approach to provide a test for the validity of the proposed hypotheses is not possible. The clinician must rely upon indirect testing. In effect, he attempts to obtain evidence that the process suggested is present by its effects rather than by sampling the involved tissues.

In the first instance, that of the 19-year-old with intra-abdominal disease, the clinician seeks bacteriologic, serologic, and roentgenologic data which support or deny the two proposed hypotheses. He searches for the effects of the suspected processes.

In the instance involving the 15-year-old boy with an intracranial mass, the available tools all provide morphologic evidence *consistent with* the hypotheses proposed. In this instance a combination of computerized axial tomography (CAT) scanning and pneumoencephalography resulted in identification of a partial mass producing internal hydrocephalus. All of the data were consistent with the presence of a pontine glioma, although a tissue diagnosis was not obtainable.

The clinician must learn to cope with indirect analysis of the patient's problems and the hypotheses developed from them. Use of morphologic and pathophysiologic knowledge will permit appropriate testing, as discussed later, in most clinical problems.

Most often the physician *samples* some aspects of the suspected pathophysiologic change in the patient. Sampling is a statistical concept based on the premise that an adequately considered portion of the whole will be representative of the whole. As used in clinical medicine the term implies a probe into either a morphologic feature *or* physiologic *or* psychologic function of the body. From such probing, inference can be made of the entire anatomic or functional unit. For example, determination of increased heart size on a roentgenogram of the chest may permit certain evaluations of cardiovascular function. Similarly, "sampling" the function of the liver by obtaining levels of bilirubin, transaminase enzymes and alkaline phosphotase permits assumption as to the physiologic state of that organ. The clinician can also utilize the Rorschach or other projective technique to gain some insight into total personality function.

As with other statistical tools, the value of sampling is limited by its adequacy. If a duodenal ulcer is suspected and an upper gastrointestinal (GI) series and barium meal examination are carried out, and only one view of the duodenum results with a suggestion of an ulcer crater, the "sample" is inadequate. Diagnostic and therapeutic conclusions may not be based upon such testing. Similarly, the elevation of serum bilirubin is inadequate to establish the state of liver cell function; one needs a larger "sample," e.g., other tests of liver function. A single abnormal response in a projective test is not an adequate basis on which to diagnose schizophrenia.

The diagnostician must satisfy the statistical criteria for appropriateness of the sample in any given instance. He is assisted in this determination by investigative criteria for diagnosis of many diseases.

Most testing of hypotheses should consist of *specific, directed questions* based upon known pathophysiologic aspects of the disease or condition suspected. The clinician wishes to know whether or not the condition suspected is present. Barring the availability of absolute criteria, the "best" answer can be found by detection of expected elements of the proposed pathophysiologic process. For example, if one suspects the presence of a collagen vascular disease such as lupus erythematosus, the presence of damage in many tissues *plus* serologic evidence of antinuclear antibody should be sought. The questions asked are related to current understanding of this disease and stem directly from its proposal as an hypothesis to explain the patient's symptoms and signs.

Specificity of diagnostic testing is the only way to insure answers directed to the hypotheses. In the section "Regularly Available Laboratory Procedures" the phenomenon of "random" search for disease will be discussed. For the purposes of the present discussions, emphasis is placed upon the necessity for having a clear question in mind whenever data are sought. One should avoid indiscriminate testing which has no question to be answered. An example may clarify this issue:

A 4-year-old female was admitted with jaundice, abdominal pain, vomiting and mild diarrhea. Examination verified the presence of jaundice, a tender, enlarged liver, and a slightly enlarged spleen. Under consideration were (1) the various forms of viral hepatitis, (2) infectious mononucleosis and (3) poisoning with liver dysfunction. The following tests were ordered: (1) hemoglobin level, (2) hematocrit, (3) red blood cell count, (4) white blood cell (WBC) count, (5) differential count, (6) platelet count, (7) complete coagulation profile, (8) urinalysis, (9) cultures of the throat, urine and stool, (10) chest X-ray, (11) electrocardiogram, (12) blood urea nitrogen, (13) glucose level, (14) serum bilirubin, (15) serum glutamic oxaloacetic transaminase level, (16) serum pyruvic transaminase, (17) alkaline phosphatase, (18) cephalin flocculation test, (19) thymol turbidity, (20) heterophile titer, (21) serum albumin/globulin ratio, (22) total serum protein, (23) serum immunoglobulin levels, (24) serum calcium level, (25) serum magnesium level, (26) serum phosphorus level, (27) serum sodium, chloride, CO_2 and potassium levels, (28) urinary and stool urobilinogen, (29) Coombs' test. . . .

The actual list was longer, but this sample illustrates the point. For many of the tests (3, 6, 7, 9, 10, 11, 12, 13, 24, 25, 26, 27 and 29) there was no clinical question to be answered.

The particular physician could not supply questions that were being asked for these tests. The search was obviously random, disorganized, wasteful, costly and unnecessary.

THE VALUE OF SPECIFIC HYPOTHESES

It should be obvious that sound practice in testing hyptheses is solidly grounded in the expression of those hypotheses. Cerebral space-occupying lesion is less apt to lead to specific diagnostic sampling than is subdural hematoma or suspected meningioma. The degree to which an hypothesis can be as narrowly constructed as possible from the data available is the degree to which specificity of testing can be applied. If the questions framed from the hypotheses are too broad, the answers received will not always be helpful. On the other hand, too narrow a construction given to hypotheses may lead to questions whose answers are so limited as to be equally nonhelpful. In forming the questions to be asked in the testing of hypotheses, one should be guided by the following principle: The data provided from testing should be directed to determining the truth or validity of the hypotheses. An example will illustrate this principle:

A 4-year-old girl presented with moderate diarrhea for 4 days. She was well until the onset of abdominal discomfort which then was followed by 4 days of copious watery stools (10 to 12/day). She became anorexic and for 3 days has refused any solid food, drinking only water and dilute 7-Up. During the past 36 hours she has become very weak and has barely been able to help her parents move her, dress her or otherwise care for her needs. The rest of the history was normal.

Physical examination revealed a sallow, pale 4-year-old who could not resist passive movements of all major muscle groups. She was mildly dehydrated as judged by dry mucus membranes and decreased skin turgor. Apart from these findings her examination was otherwise normal. Only one of several examiners felt that her abdomen was tender and that her bowel sounds were hyperactive.

The initial physician established the following hypotheses: (1) gastroenteritis, probably viral, based upon duration, character of stools, and paucity of physical findings; (2)

dehydration, based upon mucous membrane and skin findings plus historical evidence of fluid loss and probable inadequate intake; and (3) possible electrolyte imbalance believed to be a loss of all elements, based on statistical probability.

He then proceeded to test these hypotheses and discovered that (1) she had profound hypokalemia with milder hyponatremia, and (2) as judged by her failure to urinate, her high hematocrit and blood urea nitrogen, and her weight gain upon rehydration, she was felt to be 10% dehydrated. The muscle weakness was then explained (belatedly) on the basis of hypokalemia. Further, she was found to have shigellosis, which is associated with hypokalemia on occasion.

This example illustrates the necessity for drawing hypotheses broadly enough to represent the questions raised by the patient's problem. Muscle weakness should have been encompassed by the questions. Less obvious examples abound in clinical practice. It is difficult to set hypotheses broadly enough to obtain definitive answers and not so broad as to provide vague and nonspecific results. The question should be asked, "What needs to be known in this patient to provide enough information to allow as specific a therapeutic action as is possible?" In the child with gastroenteritis the answer to this question would be whether or not she had a treatable etiology to her gastroenteritis; i.e., did she have bacillary dysentry? and, also, what caused her profound weakness?

REGULARLY AVAILABLE LABORATORY PROCEDURES

The laboratory provides an array of hematologic, chemical, immunologic, bacteriologic and special techniques. Selection among the choices available is usually strictly within the clinician's initiative. He can choose narrowly or broadly and, for most tests, at will. There is a growing sentiment, both without and within medicine, that such latitude has been responsible for the escalating costs of medical care. Indiscriminate and excessive use of testing has been cited as one of the major unchecked items in medical care today.

Much of this criticism is warranted. Mindless, routine, uncertain or insecure medical practice often results in the excessive use of laboratory and other procedures. If every physician narrowed his testing to those questions that derived from his data (therefore from his hypotheses), a great number of procedures would be eliminated, and the results would not be missed at all. Many studies have demonstrated the unnecessary nature of much of what is ordered from the clinical laboratory and radiology services. One of the more devastating comments on mindless medicine derives from the observation in one hospital that much of what was ordered was not even noticed by the physician ordering it. Even abnormal results that were related to necessary therapeutic decisions were often ignored! It appeared as if the physician had completed some ritual with the ordering of the laboratory procedure and was really not interested in the result.

This error can be avoided if careful thought is centered on the patient's problems, if those questions are asked of the laboratory that are pertinent to decision making, if "routines" of ordering laboratory procedures are kept to the minimum required by sound medical practice, and if the results of one test (or tests) are noted before additional ones are sought.

The following typical clinical problem will explore the different ways of approaching laboratory diagnosis:

A 3-year-old child develops severe coughing following 3 days of upper respiratory catarrhal symptoms and signs. With the onset of fever he is brought to your attention. Examination reveals a rapid respiratory rate, fever (102° F), little or no respiratory distress, clear rhinorrhea and diffuse inspiratory rales throughout both lung fields.

A large number of children in the community have febrile respiratory disease. There is nothing in this child's previous or current history to suggest any serious underlying problem or unusual disease.

A typical approach might be to obtain a nasopharyngeal culture, chest X-ray and WBC count and administer penicillin by injection, with a prescription for oral penicillin to follow. The hypotheses upon which this course of action is based are that the child has (1) an upper respiratory infection, initially viral, ?bacterial at present, and (2) a superimposed pneumonia, probably bronchopneumonic in distribution and pneumococcal. The rationale for each test then follows: the nasopharyngeal culture, to detail pathogenic bacteria; the chest X-ray, to confirm bronchopneumonia; the WBC count, to confirm bacterial etiology; the course of penicillin, to treat suspected pneumococcal etiology. At first analysis this may seem to be an eminently sensible approach. The difficulty is that much of the reasoning is fallacious. First, the epidemiologic statistics favor a viral pneumonia by a factor of 10 or more. Second, the bacterial contents of the nasopharynx cannot be used as a guide to the etiology of the pneumonia, even if it is bacterial. Third, except in extreme cases the WBC count will not be helpful in distinguishing viral from bacterial causes of respiratory disease. Lastly, the administration of penicillin has no sound basis for all of the reasons listed above. Further, if given to this child unnecessarily, the small risk of establishing hypersensitivity looms as a major deterrent to its use.

At best one might argue that the WBC count could have been obtained, and if it is "normal" (i.e., not increased above 10,000 total cells/cw mm and not with a predominant polymorphonuclear count), the child should not be treated. If the count is abnormally high, a culture of the *blood*, not the nasopharynx, is indicated, and therapy can be pursued.

In patients almost identical to the one presented above, one will witness the following range of actions taken:

1. Hospitalization with the ordering of such tests as blood gases, multiple cultures, a complete blood count, and chest X-ray, all of which, including the hospitalization, are probably unnecessary. In addition, therapy might include a croup tent, hydration (even to the point of intravenous fluids), pulmonary physical therapy and antibiotics. Again, all of these are unnecessary.
2. Continual outpatient care with much of the same battery of laboratory tests and with a therapy which might include a succession of antibiotics.
3. Reassurance and symptomatic therapy including increased fluid intake and antipyretics with arrangements for careful follow-up.

The difference in these approaches is based largely upon the degree to which the clinician bases his judgement upon careful thought. A common statement made by some is, "I always hospitalize all children with pneumonia" or similar expressions of "routines" which substitute for thought.

A careful construction of hypotheses with precise testing and action based upon them will always stand up to rigorous analysis. "Routine" approaches seldom do, and mindless ones never can.

Selection of laboratory tests should be based upon adequate analysis of the pathophysiologic process. If acute glomerular disease is suspected from the data, the search for chemical and urinary reflection of this process can be precise. On the other hand, if one simply says "renal disease," precision is lost and selectivity is hampered. With the availability of more and more sophisticated tests and virtually no restriction on their application, selectivity becomes our only safeguard against waste.

SPECIAL LABORATORY TESTING

Special laboratory procedures include those which are costly, involve some risk to the patient other than venipuncture or similar sampling, or which are elaborate and consume technical time. Most laboratories today place restrictions on the ordering of those tests, requiring some justification and the concurrence of the director of the laboratory or his designee, frequently a clinical pathologist. Almost always, these special procedures provide results which are elaborations upon simpler determinations. Therefore, their ordering implies prior results which indicate their need. Justification should be based upon compatible clinical data plus preliminary testing which is positive. None of these should be performed in the absence of clear-cut clinical indications. For example, the anxious teenager with no findings, or the hyperactive child, or the "nervous" adult becomes the subject of elaborate thyroid diagnosis. These types of clinical situations are unaccompanied by symptoms or signs of thyroid disease, save for anxiety; there is no rationale for pursuit of tests of thyroid function. Thyroid evaluation also has been pursued frequently in lethargic or hypoactive states not even remotely related to thyroid disease.

Many examples can be found of the improper use of the clinical laboratory. It does little good to harp upon these examples and preach rectitude. What is important for our discussion is the thoughtful selective use of laboratory studies to confirm a hypothesis based solidly on clinical data.

REGULARLY AVAILABLE ROENTGENOLOGIC STUDIES

Use of roentgenologic techniques provides a valuable dimension to our diagnostic ability. Lesion localization and, to some extent, characterization can result from correct roentgenologic examination. Diseases of the cranial vault, the thorax, the abdomen, the skeleton and some of the soft tissues are most readily detected by this technique. If one's hypothesis includes an anatomic supposition in these areas, or a pathophysiologic one based on structural relationships, such roentgenologic study can often provide precise answers. Two cautions: (1) Not all anatomic or structural physiologic processes can be detected at all stages of the disease, and (2) the result of the examination may be less than is needed for convincing proof of the hypothesis. Both of these cautions apply to the rejection of an hypothesis because of absence of, or minimal changes in, the structures examined. The patient may still have the suspected process, but it remains undetected or unconfirmed by the examination.

The potential for abuse of this form of testing is enormous. Various roentgenologic examinations lend themselves to routine use, even though the result of the examination cannot provide the answers desired; e.g., routine chest roentgenogram, examination of the skull in all head injuries, and "routine" upper GI series and barium enema in all GI complaints. The competent, conscientious radiologist is constantly attempting to reduce such misuse. Such routines often substitute for thought or data collection or knowledge.

Another form of roentgenologic abuse is the practice of ordering too many examinations. This is evident in two types of clinical situations: (1) when the clinician cannot believe or accept a negative result and (2) when an initial positive result is obtained and one wishes to "follow" the course of the lesion. Too many times, absolutely negative results are simply unacceptable to the rigid diagnostician who refuses to alter his basic premise. If he has diagnosed a duodenal ulcer, he will demonstrate it even if it means multiple examinations. There is a fine line here; in some situations such action might be necessary, particularly if the examination utilized is not of high yield for the lesion sought. There is no way to offer guidelines for these situations, since they are highly dependent upon the particular clinical facts and the particular examination.

More often an acute process or dramatic finding is identified, and too frequent examination carried out subsequently. In one instance, 5 roentgenologic examinations of a child's chest occurred in 7 days after the initial diagnosis of an uncomplicated pneumonia. The particular clinician did not examine the child but simply viewed the roentgenograms for progress. An inherent danger to this practice (apart from the lack of necessity) is overexposure to X-rays. The ease of diagnostic examination from conception to death has led to overexposure for many of our patients. A number of radiologists and clinicians have voiced concern for the effects of ionizing irradiation on the individual exposed repeatedly to diagnostic examination. Of particular concern is the effect on growing or immature structures. Although most of the evidence is reassuring in that exposure is slight, there is concern for subtle effects. And certainly, unnecessary examinations are to be avoided.

A final misuse is the overreliance on structural findings or the overinterpretation of roentgenologic changes. Often the examination is expected to produce evidence of processes it cannot detect. A similar misapplication is the broad interpretation of limited findings. The character of certain processes which are radiodense cannot be defined. Pulmonary hemorrhage, pneumonic infiltrate and malignant cellular infiltrate may be seen as similar radiodense shadows in the lungs of an individual with leukemia. The radiologist may not be able to provide a "process" diagnosis, only a morphologic one.

SPECIAL ROENTGENOLOGIC PROCEDURES

Special radiologic studies can provide anatomic clues in organs not accessible to ordinary examination. Also, some studies can provide dynamic information, such as blood flow to an organ or excretion from that organ. Functional evaluation by use of contrast media or radionuclides, the use of computerized analysis of multiple radiographic images, and the use of ultrasound and various other "new" techniques have added a dimension to hypothesis testing never before available. Again, one must clearly state the questions asked, and these must be based upon solid pathophysiologic information. As with special laboratory procedures, there is usually tighter control of these special roentgenologic studies requiring justification and concurrence of the radiologist who usually performs them.

One cogent example in this area is the use of CAT scanning. The images produced by this technique provide visualization of intracranial, intrathoracic and intra-abdominal structures never before possible.

ADDITIONAL HISTORY

Occasionally in the course of establishing hypotheses it becomes clear that the best "test" is more information. This is especially true, but not limited to, an hypothesis dealing with psychologic or psychiatric abnormalities. For example, if one considers "anxiety neurosis, depressive episode" to account for recurrent abdominal pain in a preteenager, confirmatory evidence may be obtained by repetitive or extended interviews (or both). Details of personality structure and development, of interpersonal relationships, and of reactions to life situations may emerge which formerly were not explored in the first round of data collection. This kind of testing is of critical importance in those situations in which vaulting into laboratory or other testing may be expensive or dangerous. It also is useful with some infectious disease hypotheses, when contact or epidemiologic data may pinpoint potential microbial etiology and facilitate laboratory examination by making it more precise and specific.

ADDITIONAL PHYSICAL EXAMINATION

In like fashion, additional physical examination or specific clinical diagnostic tests may become important in testing hypotheses. For example, initial data may point to a cardiovascular disorder, and the results of exercise testing on physical findings may provide dynamic information to supplement the static results of the initial examination. Or, one may detect a urinary tract infection in a young male infant that suggests observation of the urinary stream to test the hypothesis that urethral valves are present. Many such instances occur in clinical practice.

It is impossible to provide generic guidelines for every instance. Rather, the specific details of a given problem may indicate the need for redefinition or elaboration upon the original physical findings.

There should be no reluctance to reexamine a patient in the light of an hypothesis generated by the initial data. In many problems, a free flow between initial data, hypothesis, laboratory testing, reexamination and additional history occurs with great regularity. The facile clinician glides between these facets of problem solving easily.

SURGICAL PROCEDURES

Sometimes, only a surgical procedure, biopsy, laparotomy or the like can provide the definite information needed to answer questions stemming from clinical hypotheses. The decision to seek such information is usually based upon the demonstrated failure of less invasive techniques to provide definitive data. For example, in acute glomerular disease it may not be possible to discriminate between the various etiologic possibilities short of examining the glomeruli directly. Or, the exact nature of inflammatory liver disease may only be defined by histologic examination of biopsied tissue due to limits in chemical definition of specific etiology. The adequate demonstration of tracheobronchial disease or the acquisition of appropriate culture material may only be available by bronchoscopy.

By and large, surgical techniques have inherent risks from very small (such as with bone marrow aspiration) to very large (such as with craniotomy). Thus, an additional factor is present against the risk the patient incurs by undergoing the procedure. The important elements of the benefit/risk judgement are the physician's and patient's perception and acceptance of the benefit/risk ratio. The patient originally appealed to the physician for help in solving his problem. The physician has analyzed the components and has decided that among the potential alternative solutions to the formulated hypotheses, a surgical procedure (or any other procedure with risk) is advisable. Part of this decision lies in the determination of the benefits that accrue to a patient as a result of the procedure (efficiency of diagnosis and therefore therapy, savings in hospital time, relief of symptoms, less cost, etc.), as contrasted to the risks (morbidity, discomfort, cost, death, etc.). Frequently, one has to calculate the *risk* of doing nothing as a benefit. From the patient's standpoint the decision is based upon his perception and clear understanding of the physician's benefit/risk reasoning plus his measure of his own ability to withstand the procedure (physical, emotional, economic and social); some have termed this the "burden" factor. All of these physician-patient variables temper the intellectual justification for the procedure. One often concludes that the direct method of diagnosis should be utilized, only to realize that it cannot or should not be applied to this patient's problem. Thus, the problem-solving process is not confined to academic considerations of the problem but is tempered by humane, social and economic considerations applied to a specific individual. This is not an abstract, theoretical process but is one which should enter *every* decision that involves a risk to the patient.

THERAPEUTIC TRIALS

Another category of testing is the therapeutic trial. Some problems defy specific diagnosis (e.g., juvenile rheumatoid arthritis). Others cannot be diagnosed adequately in the time permitted by the course of the disease (e.g., neonatal septicemia). Still others can only be confirmed by responses to therapy, although they may be suspected on diagnostic grounds. In all of these situations the hypothesis is tested by assuming it is true and then by administering as specific a therapy as is possible to the patient. The favorable response to such therapy is putative evidence that the hypothesis was correct. *As with all such indirect proofs, the clinician can be fooled by a seeming cause-effect relationship when, in fact, temporal coincidence is operative.* One of the most common examples is the administration of an antibiotic for a presumed bacterial infection with subsequent apparent response when, in fact, the patient has a viral infection which resolves spontaneously.

Since many nonbacterial and even noninfectious diseases may resemble bacterial ones, resolution following antibiotic administration does not *prove* bacterial etiology. A striking example of this phenomenon is related in detail in Chapter 2: that of a young girl with a viral infection which resembled Rocky Mountain spotted fever whose spontaneous resolution coincided with tetracycline administration.

With this caution in mind, the clinician must, however, assume a cause-effect relationship in situations in which the therapy is sufficiently specific that spontaneous relief appears improbable. If any of the following are also present, reasonable assuredness can be converted into certainty: (1) a subsequent specific diagnosis, such as a positive blood culture; (2) overwhelming compatible nonspecific diagnostic tests which revert to normal with therapy; (3) corroborative evidence obtained from sources peripheral to the patient, e.g., therapy of arsenic poisoning with subsequent demonstration of arsenic in the material believed to have been ingested; or (4) reversion to the symptomatic state (or to signs of disease) upon withdrawal of therapy. If the problem is trivial, then minimal evidence suffices, e.g., headache → aspirin → relief → no recurrence or other symptoms. If the problem is serious or chronic or both, the corroboration must be more complete, e.g., therapeutic aspirin trial for suspected rheumatoid arthritis with relief, and subsequent course and laboratory findings consistent with the diagnosis.

An example will help illustrate the above phenomena:

A 10-year-old boy had long-standing dilatation of his intrahepatic biliary system. He developed fever and shaking chills and, apart from his large liver, had a negative physical examination. The diagnosis suspected was cholangitis with possible bacteremia. Direct confirmation might be obtained from blood cultures and/or hepatic aspiration. He was deemed too ill to undergo a transcutaneous needle aspiration, hence blood cultures were obtained and antibiotics administered; the latter were chosen on the probability of enteric organisms being responsible for the episode. He promptly defervesced, and the blood cultures were sterile. Two more episodes occurred, each time therapy was discontinued, only to be relieved by readministration of the same antibiotics.

At this point we became convinced that our hypothesis was correct, even though direct proof was lacking. Since the antibiotics we were administering were nephrotoxic, we could not continue them indefinitely. The risk/balance decision had the following elements:

1. We could reverse the symptoms by use of nephrotoxic antibiotics.
2. We did not know which of a wide variety of organisms we were treating.
3. Continued "blind" therapy could result in renal destruction.
4. An alternate, less-toxic antibiotic might be available if we knew the organism in the liver and its antibiotic sensitivity pattern.
5. The process was a chronic one and could not be cured, and therefore, antimicrobial therapy would probably be necessary for a prolonged period, if not for a lifetime.

With these considerations in mind we chose to stop current therapy and, as soon as he became febrile, performed a needle aspiration of his liver. The resultant specimen cultured an enteric organism whose sensitivity pattern led us to several less-toxic choices for future therapy. They were utilized, and the patient left the hospital and has remained afebrile and well on chronic antibiotic administration.

OBSERVATION AS A DIAGNOSTIC TEST

A final form of clinical "testing" is no test at all. There are some problems, and some situations within clinical problems, that cannot be resolved by any test. In these instances the clinician should do nothing except to observe his patient continually. The course of the disease may of itself be diagnostic, or the delay may permit definite tests to become positive. An example is the young child with undiagnosable intermittent febrile episodes. Only continued observation may provide the ultimate diagnosis of rheumatoid arthritis which, in its early stages, may only be manifested by bouts of unexplainable fever. Another example of this phenomenon is the individual with abdominal pain uncharacteristic of any single disease entity and associated with indefinite laboratory results. Only continual observation will yield the ultimate diagnosis of acute appendicitis; at a future point, definite surgery can be carried out.

The most difficult decisions in medical practice are frequently those in which the physician must choose between doing something (anything) versus doing nothing. It is very difficult to do nothing in the face of a multitude of choices, many of which are innocuous, if unrewarding, in performance or expensive to the patient. Often a physician is tempted to "do a few tests" while observing the patient. After all, he argues, "the tests can't hurt the patient, and we're waiting anyway"; such reasoning is specious, can be costly to the patient, and on occasion can produce harm. An example follows:

A 23-month-old infant was seen because of excessive irritability characterized by the drawing of her legs into her abdomen. She had no other symptoms or signs. The cautious examiner realized that the reason for her behavior could range from a trivial and perhaps undiagnosable cause to major intra-abdominal disasters. After definitely ascertaining the lack of a disease process elsewhere in the body he decided that the child should be observed in the hospital with reexamination at frequent intervals. However, he could not restrain himself from the temptation to do something. On the way to the ward he decided to obtain abdominal roentgenologic examination. The child was detained for more than 1 hour before the examination could be performed. During this interval she was attended by a nurse's aide inexperienced with young infants. The child quieted down in the X-ray corridor reassuring the aide that all was well. When the technician was ready to perform the examination, she discovered a cold, unresponsive child obviously in shock. Heroic management from that point on led to eventual recovery following definitive surgery. The child had acute appendicitis with rupture and peritonitis.

One can argue that the examination was totally justifiable. Upon analysis, however, the critical element was frequent *clinical* observation. The correct decision was to do nothing else at that point. Even an efficiently performed abdominal roentgenogram was not in order, given the physical findings. It most likely would have yielded no information. The reason it was ordered in this instance was the imperative compulsion that many experience to do something, anything instead of nothing. It's a perfectly understandable emotion in an action-oriented profession, but must be resisted when appropriate.

SUMMARY

Testing of hypotheses is often as specific as the clinical data and the specific hypothesis. It is difficult to generalize about so specific a relationship. This chapter has dealt with some of the guidelines a diagnostician may use when approaching specific diagnosis. Above all, a thoughtful approach based upon the hypothesis is stressed. Random, routine or otherwise-independent testing taken separately from the specific data is usually wasteful and unrewarding and can be risky for the patient. Finally, in some situations it may be better to do nothing at all rather than "anything."

Chapter 6

Clinical Action and Inaction

When many refer to the problem-solving process, they really refer to its final steps, to the decision-making process in therapy. The appeal of this step in the process is in its active nature, in its often definitive results and in its proximity to the popular concept of the physician as healer.

The preceding chapters have amply documented the many steps necessary in the process *prior to* therapeutic decisions. Although somewhat redundant, it must be emphasized that effective action is only possible by effective data collection, analysis, and problem solving.

"Action" implies the successful completion of the diagnostic process with selection of the most likely or the correct explanation for the patient's clinical problem. It has often been said that armed with such information a monkey would then select the correct therapy. This oversimplification is untrue. Decision making in clinical therapy involves the same reasoning ability as do the earlier steps. It is true that given an adequate diagnosis, choice of therapy in many instances is straightforward, but not always; and not always when it appears straightforward is the therapeutic decision that simple. In this chapter we will explore the major aspects of deciding what to do or not to do after the diagnostic process reaches a certain point.

INSTITUTING THERAPY

The first task in this process is to decide *when and if* to begin therapy as opposed to diagnostic procedures. Factors influencing the initiation of therapy are (1) a correct definitive diagnosis, (2) a treatable disease process, (3) the urgency of correction of pathophysiology, (4) the necessity for specific diagnosis, (5) consent of the patient and (6) the inherent risks of the particular therapy.

At some point in the analysis of a clinical illness it is obvious that therapy is to be initiated. Most frequently, this coincides with the *establishment of a diagnosis.* If specific tests have reliably indicated that one of the hypotheses considered is correct, little further need be done. Unless one is motivated by additional factors, therapy can begin as soon as this point is reached. Such additional factors might include the need to establish criteria for following the effects of therapy, the desirability of increasing some desirable host response prior to administration of therapy which will remove the stimulus to that response, the necessity for precise timing of therapy, and practical considerations involved in the safe application of therapy.

Assume a diagnosis of rheumatoid arthritis has been reasonably established in a patient. One could undertake therapy immediately, but it is preferable to measure certain serum indicators of inflammatory activity, to determine the degree of impairment of mobility and to assess physical strength. All of these will be used as long-term indicators of the progression of disease and the patient's response to therapy. Delay in therapy to permit accumulation of data is legitimate and necessary.

Some clinicians feel therapy for certain infectious diseases (such as streptococcal and pneumococcal infections of mild to moderate severity) should be slightly delayed in initiation to permit a type-specific immune response. They argue that such delay does not damage the patient but does assist in future resistance to infection with that same agent or very closely related types. Other examples of this type of reasoning are delaying surgical approach to abscess drainage (awaiting the natural walling-off effect of inflammation), delay in the operative intervention in peritonitis to allow localization, and delay in the therapy of many diseases to permit homeostatic equilibrium to be reestablished.

If therapy must be precisely tuned to some events external to the patient, it may be withheld until that timing is propitious. This is an infrequent occurrence but occasionally is necessary.

Practical considerations range from the simple to the complex. Therapy may be delayed for a variety of reasons related to the availability of the drug or technique or technician. It may be contingent upon adequate explanation to the patient or acceptance by the patient's family, and so on.

Of necessity, one must be dealing with a *treatable process*. Simple as this concept may seem, it is often abused. Therapy may be initiated in the erroneous belief that the process will respond, or with the vague hope that it will, even if the clinical facts indicate otherwise. Nothing is crueler than to employ a fruitless form of treatment which arouses false anticipation of benefit in the patient. The inevitable failure often results in depressive symptoms. One quasilegitimate use of inappropriate therapy is occasionally found in *some* terminally ill patients.

Usually, the most persuasive element in initiation of therapy is the *urgency* occasioned by the progression or stage of the disease. Thus, acute emergent or fulminant processes are treated very early in the reasoning process, often before a definitive diagnosis is established. In bacterial meningitis, therapy begins with the anatomic diagnosis and does not await specific identity of the etiologic agent. Acute hemorrhagic diseases usually demand blood, or blood component replacement, prior to the precise knowledge of etiol-

ogy. Many abdominal surgical conditions require immediate approach prior to complete definition of the problem. The list is long and the practice occurs daily.

In contrast, some disease states demand specific identification *before* therapy is instituted. The need for diagnosis usually rests on the selection of therapy, the wish to avoid the effects of too broad a therapeutic approach, or the fact that therapy may obliterate the etiologic clues without curing the patient. If premature therapy is employed in the latter situation, the physician is then confronted with a process not under control, and without knowledge of what caused it.

Often, therapy which is specific, and indicated, cannot be applied because the patient, guardians or relatives object and do not wish to give consent. The reasons range the gamut of human motivation, from fear to intelligent discrimination. Examples include religious aversion to certain therapies, such as refusal of blood administration by members of the Jehovah's Witnesses religious sect; rejection of therapeutic abortion on personal, philosophic or religious grounds; fear of surgery or anesthesia; lack of confidence in the adequacy of the physician or his efforts; fear of side effects, and the inability to accept painful, disfiguring or otherwise discomforting therapy. Medicine is not a computerized slot-machine discipline. One does not enter symptoms and signs, obtain laboratory data, establish a diagnosis, and automatically select and apply the correct therapy. The physician is dealing with people who can think and feel and, surprisingly to some physicians, have an opinion concerning their own fate.

There have been parents who have refused therapy for their children which was exceedingly dangerous or uncomfortable. There are others who refused therapy for the children on no more reason than their own stubbornness, hostility, loneliness or mental aberration. The physician faces difficult choices in situations in which indicated therapy is denied. Should he reject the patient and turn his care over to someone else? Should he reject the patient's decision and continue to care for the patient? Should he attempt to convince the patient? If so, how far should he go? Should he use fear, intimidation or other forms of coercion, or should he be patient and employ softer means? There are no universal answers to these difficult questions. All alternatives are acceptable at a societal level, although some of them are more "approved" than others. One hopes the physician is guided by sincere interest in his patient, and not in his own ego or pride, in his final choice of response.

One hesitates to recommend therapy with a high degree of inherent risk. Thus, a delay in onset of therapy may occur when potent agents or modalities are to be employed. The physician may need to solidify his diagnosis, educate and instruct his patient, prepare for the expected adverse effects, or measure certain physiologic parameters which he anticipates will be altered by the therapy.

CHOOSING AMONG ALTERNATIVE TREATMENTS

The second major task confronting the clinician is his choice of *which* therapy to utilize, assuming there are alternative forms available to him. Although seemingly simple, this choice can be quite complex. The physician must weigh (1) the pharmacology (if a drug) or the physiology (if a device or technique) of the therapeutic agent(s); (2) the toxicity, side effect or unwanted effect of the agent or modality; (3) practical consideration in delivery of the therapy to the patient; and (4) the acceptance by, and effect on, the patient.

One must always assess the effectiveness of a specific treatment in a particular patient. For drugs, such things as the size of the dose needed, the route of administration, absorption, metabolism and excretion may play a part in choice. From general information about the drug, the physician must specify for his patient. A simple example is the choice between a parenteral and oral form of penicillin in a child with proved streptococcal pharyngitis. Oral therapy must be extended over 10 days and must be given 3 to 4 times/day. It takes a certain kind of parent-child combination for the physician to be certain that therapy will be completed. Knowledge of the pharmacology of penicillin assures the physician that either mode, oral or parenteral, will provide sufficient blood and tissue levels to achieve eradication of the organism. However, he may choose the parenteral form for a parent-child configuration which is unlikely to complete oral intake. On the other hand, he may choose oral therapy for other parent-child units, based upon reliability and the cost and acceptance benefits of the oral regimen.

Many more complex situations occur in clinical practice which require astute and precise knowledge of clinical pharmacology. The therapy of the individual with asthma in acute exacerbation requires skillful use of several modalities of therapy, each of which is alterable for specific patient situations. Good practice in this area demands a pharmacologic juggling act dependent upon keen appreciation of the effects and side effects of the agents employed. Therapy other than drugs must also be assessed for each patient. If complicated maneuvers are required and home therapy must be carried out, careful assessment of the patient's temperament and abilities must be made, or a suitable substitute selected. If equipment is involved, its use and maintenance are factors that enter the decision.

This discussion is not intended to be exhaustive in terms of all possible modes of therapy. That is impossible. But common to all selection decisions is individual assessment of how that particular therapy fits in with this particular patient. It makes little difference if it is digitalis, physical therapy or a surgical procedure that is being assessed. The issues involved in the choice are identical; their value may differ from modality to modality and from patient to patient. The constant and overriding question is, "What is best for this patient, given his disease and personal characteristics?"

In general, in choosing among alternatives, that therapy is selected which is the most specific available, the easiest to administer and accept, associated with the least side effects, the cheapest and the most realistic. All of these features may not be present in the single mode of therapy. Individual assessment must be made.

LONG-RANGE ASPECTS OF THERAPEUTIC DECISIONS

A third major consideration in therapeutic decision making is the long-range prospects of the clinical condition treated. In many clinical situations, the choice of initial therapy is conditioned by the knowledge of the natural progress of the disease process. For example, in acute angioneurotic edema, therapy can be selected which is applied over a short time, and little consideration of long-range administration need be tendered. Thus, epinephrine and aminophylline may be employed with little regard to long-term effects. However, with chronic forms of urticaria one would be loathe to expose the patient to prolonged use of these agents, and different therapeutic modalities are chosen.

This consideration will hold sway in most chronic conditions. Diabetes, rheumatoid arthritis, asthma, chronic pulmonary diseases, chronic pyelonephritis, chronic hepatitis, chronic psychologic disorders and many others require a long view before any therapy is initiated. What will suffice for the acute manifestations cannot always be employed on a chronic basis. Frequently, this fact will force the physician to choose an alternate, less efficacious therapy but one with the potential for tolerance over the long haul. An excellent example is found in the therapy of rheumatoid arthritis. Corticosteroids are potent anti-inflammatory agents in this disorder. Acetylsalicylic acid is less potent but still efficacious. It, rather than steroids, is the therapy of choice because the clinician realizes that therapy will be prolonged, perhaps for a lifetime. Aspirin therapy avoids the inevitable consequences of the side effects of long-term steroid therapy's growth failure, steroid diabetes, myopathies, etc.

SELECTING THERAPY FOR THE "WHOLE" PATIENT

A fourth general consideration is the overall health of the patient. The setting in which the current problem occurs is often an overriding consideration in therapeutic selection. It is one thing to treat pneumonia in an otherwise healthy young adult, and quite another to treat the same disease in a child with chronic cardiovascular, metabolic or pulmonary conditions. It is yet another to treat pneumonia in a child who either has a disease, or treatment, which results in immunosuppression. In each of these instances the

therapeutic decisions are quite different despite the fact that the acute disease being treated is identical.

It is not only concomitant disease that alters therapeutic decisions, but therapy the patient is receiving. Drug antagonism, or synergistic side effects, may limit the physician's options. A patient receiving digitalis should not receive agents which will lower serum and tissue potassium, as this will potentiate digitalis side effects. In general, patients receiving a bactericidal antibiotic should not receive a bacteriostatic one in addition, as drug antagonism is a possibility. Patients receiving drugs which reduce the neutrophile population should not subsequently be given another agent which does the same thing. In today's clinical practice, with its multiple pharmacopeia for many patients, such opportunities for adverse drug interactions abound. I encountered one recent patient in her sixth month of pregnancy who was receiving eight different drugs, *plus* those she was taking as home remedies. Apart from the potential effects on her fetus, the opportunities for adverse reactions in the light of her altered physiology were enormous. The drugs had been prescribed by four different physicians, none of whom appeared to take into account the therapy for her other ailments. One cannot afford, for the patient's sake, to practice such willy-nilly therapeutics. Sound medical practice demands that therapeutic decisions take into account all factors in the patient to whom the therapy is directed.

DECIDING NOT TO TREAT AND THE USE OF "PLACEBO" THERAPY

A final consideration is that sometimes *no* therapy should be given. Inaction is as positive a decision as selection of some action. For diagnostic tests, as well as therapy, the same rules apply. Don't do anything that is not necessary. Don't administer treatment to your patient solely for the sake of doing something.

If the diagnostic process produces an answer for which there is no therapy, none should be given. For example, the diagnosis of recurrent herpes simplex infection may be made in an 18-year-old woman. Nothing is indicated. Vitamins B_{12}, B_6, and the B complex, ether topically, smallpox vaccination, *Lactobacillus acidophilus* orally, a variety of local creams and lotions—all have been employed in this frustrating, inconvenient and painful disease. All of these treatments have been applied with the same result—they are no better than nothing. Yet the temptation is great. The patient is uncomfortable, the physician is anxious to help, the relatives stand by impatiently—all factors pressuring the physician to act. If the physician is certain there is no therapy for the disease in question, he should tell the patient just that. Neither the physician nor the patient should be deluded into false hopes by the employment of an unnecessary therapy or nostrum. There are limits to the ability to heal which all physicians must acknowledge.

The physician must learn to accept such therapeutic impotence with grace and equanimity. In addition, he has an obligation to transmit this information to his patient in an effort to prevent, or limit, the seeking of "help" elsewhere. A good doctor-patient relationship will permit such decisions to be received with confidence.

If the physician is in doubt as to the value of reported treatments, he can seek out definitive information himself or obtain reliable, mature consultation. Details concerning these modes of obtaining information beyond the physician's base of knowledge will differ from problem to problem. What is important is that the physician seeks the information if he is unsure. Doing so can result in saving the patient the risk of unnecessary, and possibly dangerous, therapy.

There are additional reasons for clinical inaction, apart from untreatable conditions. On occasion the indicated therapy is simply inappropriate for the patient (as has been discussed previously). Or the patient may have legitimate reasons for refusing to accept the therapy. Or the physician, the patient, or both may decide the process is not significant enough to warrant therapy. This is an extremely personal equation which will differ from individual to individual. One patient with recurrent staphylococcal furunculosis will accept a rigid and compulsive personal cleanliness regimen. Another will decide the problem is simply not that troublesome to require such a change in life routine. One

patient with chronic pain will refuse elaborate, costly and dangerous therapeutic measures and tolerate the discomfort. Another with seemingly less pain will accept any therapeutic modality that promises relief regardless of the elaborateness, cost or danger. In fact, pain and other forms of discomfort afford the best examples of individual variation, tolerance and acceptance or resistance to therapy. There simply are some individuals who, having sought help for some discomforting symptom complex, will not accept the recommended treatment when they weigh it on their own personal balance. The wise clinician learns to recognize and accept such judgements, even if it means he will do nothing for the patient.

As this book is being written the news broadcasts are reporting a young father in Ohio who has decided to disconnect himself from his hemodialysis unit. This action will insure his death from chronic renal failure. He has decided that the therapy is not worth it—despite the fact that the alternative is death. Most young or inexperienced physicians, and some experienced ones, cannot understand such motivation. After all, they reason, if there is a treatment, it must be better than death. Not for everyone. We do not all march to the same drummer. Of course, this discussion does not refer to the irrational, or suicidal, or temporary decisions that many patients make which almost mandate active resistance by the physician. A fine sense of discrimination must be exercised to distinguish the two types of refusal to accept therapy.

The discussion has not taken into account that the personal code of some physicians will not permit them to accept such patient decisions under any circumstances. One example of this is the physician who obtained a court order permitting him to conduct a surgical procedure on an infant with intestinal obstruction and Down's syndrome. He could not accept the parents' decision to allow the child to die by denying permission for surgery. There are many such examples in medicine. The recent debate on abortion has clearly cast light on the differing attitudes of physicians and laity alike about the "rights" of the various parties involved.

In most of these situations we are in areas

in which society has not established binding guidelines. A great deal of latitude is permitted patient and physician in choosing among widely divergent alternatives. The aspiring physician must discover for himself the particular niche he will occupy in these ethical and moral dilemmas. It is a very uncomfortable process for some who would prefer fixed guidelines and a rigid code where there are none.

To the author, it appears that society is wise not to legislate certain moral and ethical issues, since individuals have such varying personal philosophies, religious convictions, and values. To fix any one set of rules on the public at large is bound to infringe on personal rights for large segments of our population. Similarly, physicians would be constrained to act in ways that are repugnant to their personal ethics. Rather, each physician in combination with his patient must find that level within permissible behavior at which they wish to operate. There will always be difficult and uncomfortable situations in a free society which has chosen not to set fixed guidelines in certain human activities. As long as this remains so, the mature physician will be measured by the degree to which he recognizes this phenomenon, searches his own soul and develops a personal code of behavior and a sensitivity to that of his patient's.

"Placebo" therapy is a special instance of the no therapy concept. In this instance, instead of rejecting any form of therapy, the physician employs a supposedly innocuous treatment unrelated to the condition being treated. Many physicians employ such substances as vitamins, lactic acid and glucose in clinical situations in which they feel no specific therapy is indicated. However, they are reluctant to prescribe nothing for a patient whom they estimate requires some therapeutic intervention to maintain doctor-patient confidence. In some situations, placebo therapy is employed to sustain the patient in a more significant diagnostic or therapeutic relationship; in others, to prevent the patient from seeking dubious nonmedical intervention. To many, these are examples of legitimate exercise of the placebo concept. The slight "sin" of using false therapy is overcome by the greater "good" of the sustained bene-

fits of the continuing relationship between the doctor and the patient.

There are many current critics of the practice of placebo administration. The most extreme argue that it is, at best, a deceptive practice and, at worst, an evil practice. Such critics cite the substitution of placebo therapy for psychologic or psychiatric therapy, the use of placebos as a form of disdain for the patients intelligence, the laziness implied in the administration of a useless remedy, the dangers inherent in some forms of placebo medication, and the false hopes aroused by the administration of a seemingly beneficial treatment. These characteristics of some of the practices utilizing the placebo concept are felt to be examples of unsound, and even unethical, medical practice.

As with many such controversies in clinical medicine, the truth appears to lie between the extremes. There are legitimate clinical circumstances, in the author's view, for use of the placebo concept, such as those cited initially. However, there exists a number of abuses and misuses of placebo administration, which the critics have identified. It appears sound to accept the legitimate usage while rejecting the abuses.

Placebo therapy should never substitute for considered thought in the care of patients. Placebos ought not be given as replacement for counseling or psychiatric treatment. Placebos should not be a form of intellectual snobbery on the physician's part, in effect proving that the patient is an inferior being because he can be "fooled" by sugar pills. And obviously the use of placebos should not be a financial device to continue contact with a patient who otherwise does not require any medical care.

RISK/BENEFIT DECISION MAKING

One consideration inherent in therapeutic decision making is the concept of risk/benefit to the patient. It is such an important aspect of problem solving and decision making as to deserve separate discussion.

For each set of problem/solution configurations there are benefits and risks to the patient. There is no convincing example that is free of this balance. From the simplest disease/therapy situations to the most complex, such a ratio exists. It is not always voiced, but it is an integral part of a physician's behavior.

The first factor to be considered is the risk of the disease or condition. In general, but not always in the specific case, this risk determines subsequent actions. For a patient with meningococcemia and septic shock the risk of death is high, conditioning both the speed and quality of therapeutic action. In like fashion, but not as obvious and infrequently analyzed, the individual with an acute headache has minimal risk of a serious process. This fact similarly conditions the physician's response. In general, diseases with maximal risk in terms of morbidity and mortality allow the selection of therapy, which can range from the least to the most beneficial, almost without regard to the hazards of such therapy. Conversely, diseases with minimal risk inherently require a high order of benefit and virtually no hazard in the therapy selected. Some examples might illustrate this point more clearly. A patient with an inaccessible brainstem tumor might be treated blindly with potent irradiation despite low benefit yield and high potential for adverse consequences. A patient with a lipoma of the subcutaneous tissues of the arm should never be treated with such blindness and potency. The risks from the lesion obviously do not justify it. But what of the following examples?

> A young male adult had moderately severe abdominal pain and gastrointestinal hemorrhage culminating in a diagnosis of severe bleeding duodenal ulcer. What level of therapy is justified? A modest medical regimen including diet and drugs, or immediate surgery?
>
> A 35-year-old woman had a carcinoma of the breast diagnosed without any evidence of spread. Should she have the mass removed, or be irradiated? Or should she undergo simple or radical mastectomy with or without irradiation?
>
> These questions cannot be answered simply and opinions differ depending upon the interpretations of the benefit/risk ratio in each instance.

The risk of the disease alone does not always fix the level of therapy. The benefit to be derived from a given modality weighs heavily in the decision, as does the risk inherent in the therapy. Most often the benefit/ risk ratio is thought of strictly in terms of the therapy itself. Actually the process blends the risks from the disease with the benefits and risks from the therapy.

Virtually every therapeutic modality has some inherent risk. Almost anything that is done or given to a patient has the potential for causing some harm. Some of the risk is intrinsic to the therapy—there is no way in which inhalation anesthesia sufficient for surgical therapy can be administered to thousands of persons without a few suffering adverse consequences, even death. Some risk comes about not because of a high potential intrinsic to the therapy, but because the patient is unusually responsive to some action of the agent. During the height of the several influenza epidemics in the past several decades, aspirin was administered to hundreds of thousands of patients; many bled from the expected gastric irritation, a few had severe coagulation disturbances, and a rare individual experienced an idiosyncratic severe reaction to this seemingly innocuous agent. Similarly, in some patients, aspirin produces severe bronchospasm resembling allergic asthma. The risk is present in almost every action taken. It must be assessed to the extent known *prior to* recommending a particular therapy and again *during* the course of therapy.

There is the risk of doing nothing. When it is decided that no therapy is justified, the risk of the disease becomes paramount, without modifying influence. In all situations in which therapy is not recommended, the risk from the disease must be estimated.

How does the clinician utilize this information? It would be very satisfying and comforting to report that these formulae can be applied with mathematical precision. However, gaps in our information, the varying assessment of benefit and risk, the subjective nature of the patient's and physician's definitions of benefit and risk, the unknowable individual variation in reactivity to therapy— all prevent methodical employment of structured ratios. At best we employ the average risk and average benefit, modified by those *known* circumstances of disease and patient variation. A *judgement* is made. Surgery for this condition in this patient is justified because . . . , whereas surgery for the same condition in this other individual is not justified because. . . .

It should always be remembered that the risks spoken of so lightly by the physician are experienced *by the patient*. George Bernard Shaw summed up this fact in *The Doctor's Dilemma*.

Too often physicians behave as if the risk were being applied theoretically. The personal nature of the risk cannot be forgotten. It applies to people. People get drug reactions. People die from anesthesia, or surgery, or drugs. People die from diseases unrecognized or improperly treated. Some years ago a young intern developed staphylococcal furunculosis, as did many of his peers. He was given chloramphenicol (in those days there was little concern for the toxicity of this drug and great admiration for its effectiveness). The infection cleared rapidly but the intern awoke one morning with urticaria, fever, an oppressive feeling in his chest, and massive apprehension. He was told that he had a reaction to chloramphenicol. The attending physician at the intern's bedside said in a bemused way, "I've never had that happen to me before." The intern realized then, and retained the realization thereafter, that it didn't happen to him (the physician), it happened to the intern! Abed for 5 days with shaking chills, fever, severe itching and urticaria, profound lethargy, anorexia and malaise, the intern recognized that what was a statistic to the physician was a horror to him, the patient. All of us need not experience therapeutic misadventures to become sensitive to the personal nature of risk, although some have suggested that physicians who have been patients make better doctors! We only need to have our interpersonal antennae tuned always to the patient, not to the disease or the diagnostic test or the therapy, but to the human being with whom the physician is interacting. "Medicine," "disease," "treatment"—all are personal; they occur in and are placed upon people. This fact should never be forgotten.

CONTINUAL PROBLEM SOLVING IN CLINICAL PRACTICE

Another important factor in clinical management and problem solving is the continuous nature of the process. Once the physician has completed the intellectual maneuvers required in diagnosis, selection and initiation of treatment, he cannot banish the episode from existence. The process is continual, as the effects of therapy, the effects of the disease as it comes under control, the complications, the residue, the unwanted side effects of therapy, and the patient's response are all gauged.

The significance of continuous care and evaluation is evident in simple as well as complex problems. The individual who presents with straightforward streptococcal pharyngitis requires continuous vigilance on the part of the physician. Is the therapy adequate? Is the penicillin taken? Has the streptococcus been eradicated? Have any contacts been infected? An entire series of clinical problems stem from a simple "strep" throat. Inadequate clinical care would be involved if any of these questions were not asked. Similarly, a "routine" urinary tract infection probably involves a lifelong (the patient's lifetime) quest for continuing disease. Since many individuals initially infected become chronically infected, both diagnostic and therapeutic problem solving continues. Except for relatively few acute problems, most pathophysiologic processes require thought beyond the acute episode, often for weeks or months, and sometimes for the rest of the patient's life.

The initiation of therapy, therefore, may only be an intermediary step in the problem-solving process for the individual patient. Many clinicians have attempted to recognize this fact in their practices with various devices to insure follow-up care and evaluation automatically. Others develop a longitudinal work sheet with designated routine points and space to insert unexpected or untoward events. Whatever the technique, the importance of follow-up cannot be underestimated.

THE FACTUAL KNOWLEDGE OF THE PHYSICIAN AS A FACTOR IN THERAPY

Other considerations in therapeutic decision making are similar or identical in principle to those previously detailed for diagnoses. One of these deserves reconsideration as it applies to therapy, particularly drug therapy. The factual knowledge possessed by the physician is a critical factor in intelligent therapeutic problem solving. It is the data on which he will judge selection of therapy, benefit to the patient, and risk. We have detailed the methods used to acquire such information (see Chapter 3). There are some general rules that each physician should apply to the therapy he utilizes.

1. For every therapy recommended, the physician should know or acquire the basic information needed **before** *he recommends it for a single patient.*

This principle is amply illustrated in the use of antibiotics. The first disasters recorded for chloramphenicol were among children of physicians. The doctor-parents administered this potent drug to their children following receipt of samples for clinical trials. For the most part they were unfamiliar with its potential for toxicity. Despite such precedent, even today, physicians do not hesitate to administer the "latest" antibiotic without precise knowledge of its pharmacology. They do so despite the fact that they have available, and have used successfully, adequate antibiotics for the infectious diseases occurring in their patients.

Students are in a unique position in that they have not developed their therapeutic habits. Therefore, they can learn to apply this principle. In antibiotic therapy this would result in no more than six agents for you to be familiar with in ambulatory practice and two or three additional ones for the occasional patient with more severe disease requiring hospitalization. Contrast this with the practice of one physician in which *nine* separate antibiotics were used to treat "sore throats" in his patients. As you progress in your knowledge of clinical pharmacology, you will learn that a relatively limited range of drugs is required for the bulk of your practice. The clinical pharmacology of each of them should be learned until it can be recited at will. Then, and only then, can the physician evaluate each new agent introduced. If only a minor change in formulation is introduced, there is little need to substitute it for the established therapy. Only if the new drug *significantly* changes efficacy, or lessens toxicity, or in some other way offers a major advantage beyond what can now be accom-

plished, should that drug be included in the array of agents available to the physician.

It is inexcusable to administer to a patient any agent with which the physician is totally unfamiliar. There simply is no excuse for such irrational action. The inherent risks are magnified if the physician is unaware of them and if the patient receiving the agent has some feature which would have caused the physician to recognize the potential sensitivity. The practice of sending physicians samples and of gaudy, impressive advertising has increased the temptation to try a recently introduced drug without proper knowledge of its clinical pharmacology.

2. Clinical pharmacology should be learned and applied.

In some ways a restatement of the previous principle, this recommendation focuses attention on some specific aspects of drug therapy. With the plethora of agents available, and with multiple drug use common and often indicated, the opportunities for drug interaction of unwanted nature have increased. For drugs that are commonly employed in tandem, it is essential that their interaction with one another be known. It is not an uncommon occurrence to encounter in a clinical situation the failure of a drug therapy which should have resulted in success. Such failures are frequently the result of cancelation, or reduction, of the effect of one drug administered by another. Or side effects may be potentiated, or the desired effect may be magnified beyond desirable limits. The disease process may be accentuated by inappropriate use of certain agents in certain conditions. The hazards of drug utilization are many and varied. Only the physician who is knowledgeable in current clinical pharmacology can avoid them or minimize their effect.

There are other aspects of pharmacology which have very practical consequences. Knowledge of the relationship between maturing or inducible enzyme systems and drug metabolism frequently permits greater, or demands lesser, latitude in the application of certain agents. Knowledge of excretion routes and their significance can facilitate use of drugs for certain organ-localized disease and prohibit use in renal or liver failure. Knowledge of drug metabolism can assist in alteration of drug dosage in diseases likely to impair breakdown.

3. The list of usable therapeutic agents and modalities should be kept to a minimum.

Although use of a wide variety of chemotherapeutic agents and other therapy is superficially attractive, the wise clinician will narrow his choice for each usage to one, or a few, treatment regimens with which he can become thoroughly familiar. Familiarity means fewer mistakes in application, more rapid recognition and therapy of side effects, greater flexibility in adjustment of the therapy to individual situations, and a better opportunity to grasp clinical pharmacology thoroughly. Earlier, antibiotic administration was utilized in illustration of a similar point. The physician who has solid command of a relatively few antibiotics can serve all of his patients' needs intelligently and thoroughly. The dilettante who dispenses a multitude of drugs rarely knows them well and is either surprised by their effects or, worse, remains ignorant of them. Such careless usage is to be deplored.

4. "Fads" in therapy should be avoided.

Alexander Pope's advice is the most sensible in this regard; in *An Essay on Criticism*, he states:

> "Be not the first by whom the new are tried,
> Nor yet the last to lay the old aside."

This is a concise statement of sound judgement. Too often, physicians seize the opportunity afforded by the introduction of new compounds on the market. Only later is it discovered that the new agent offers no real benefits and, in fact, has disturbing side effects.

One should not, however, be the last to accept and utilize a really significant new introduction. The soundest advice is to follow the progress of the new agent in the specialty journals and await the expert opinion that the agent has achieved its niche in sound clinical practice.

5. Continuous control should be exercised over any therapeutic regimen prescribed. Patients receive medication(s) even for the simplest of complaints. When such usage is justifiable, the physician's responsibility does not end with the prescription. Careful and continuous follow-up with monitoring of both drug effect and side effects is essential.

6. Discontinuation of therapy may be the wisest choice in certain clinical circumstances.

Most clinicians learn that a given course of therapy is indicated for a certain condition. Thus, once diagnosed, that condition is remedied by prescribing the given course in its entirety. There are a number of reasons to retract therapy in such circumstances:

1. Failure of effect.
2. A superimposed condition contradicts use of currently advised therapy. For example, for a patient given steroid cream for contact dermatitis who then develops a local pyogenic infection, the steroid should be discontinued until the infection is appropriately treated.
3. Any significant adverse effect.
4. The original diagnosis is in error.
5. The original diagnosis is in question. An example of this is the patient suspected of having bacterial meningitis whose laboratory values subsequently indicate clearly that this is an episode of aseptic meningitis. In this circumstance one need not continue with the prescribed 10 to 21 days of antibiotics.
6. More effective therapy can now be given.
7. Equally, or even slightly less effective, therapy can now be given more safely or by a more acceptable route.

Despite what are seemingly obvious reasons for discontinuation of therapy, many clinicians cling to an original regimen because completion is so ingrained in our therapeutic application. Too often a child suspected of streptococcal pharyngitis has oral penicillin therapy initiated, and 10 days completed, despite the lack of convincing confirmatory evidence.

One sure method for at least reminding the physician of the need for assessment of therapy is the prescription of less than a full course at the outset. The necessity to reorder or rewrite a prescription will serve as a timely jog to the memory to reevaluate the need.

SUMMARY

This chapter has dealt with clinical action and inaction. It has been pointed out that the problem-solving process does not end with diagnosis but continues even beyond therapy. Some clues as to the rationale of therapeutic decision making and specific advice for good practice and habit with avoidance of error have been presented.

Chapter 7

The Pediatric Emergency and Clinical Problem Solving

INTRODUCTION

I've elected to approach this and subsequent specific clinical chapters with a case-oriented approach. Standard textbooks will detail the types and varieties of conditions contained within each category. I am attempting to define and analyze with you the problem-solving approach that is generic to any specific condition within the given chapter categorical title.

For pediatric emergencies, I've chosen three cases from my own experience.

Case #1. A 4-month-old child presents with fever for 2 days, rhinorrhea, and progressive lethargy with very recent onset of lack of response to external stimuli. Physical examination reveals an hypotonic infant unresponsive to pain, areflexic, cyanotic and pale, with a thin, threading pulse of 150/min, respirations of 10/min, a blood pressure of 60/0, and a rectal temperature of 104° F (39.5° C). Rapid examination fails to reveal any other gross abnormalities.

Case #2. A 2-year-old is rushed into the emergency room, vomiting blood. The child was well until 1 hour ago, when he was discovered with his mother's pregnancy pills, containing iron and vitamins, strewn about him on the bathroom floor. He is lethargic and unresponsive with the following vital signs: blood pressure, 50/0; respiratory rate, 30/min; pulse rate, 160/min; and temperature, 96° F. Rapid physical examination reveals no significant abnormalities.

Case #3. A 6-year-old fell from a tree in his back yard. When discovered, minutes later, he was confused, apathetic, and began making uncontrollable jerking movements of his arms and legs, lapsed into unconsciousness with his eyes "rolled back into his head," and bit his tongue. He was rushed to the hospital, at which time his examination revealed a semicomatose child responsive only to loud or painful stimuli, with weakness of his left arm and leg, increased tendon reflexes in the left but no other positive physical findings. The right side of his scalp was dirty and grass was evident in his hair overlying a 2-cm, soft, fluctuant mass beneath his scalp.

CASE ANALYSIS

Each of these children represents commonly encountered pediatric emergencies. The purpose of this chapter is to explore the *thinking* involved in emergency care for infants and children rather than to provide a cookbook method for a series of emergencies. There are other texts to accomplish the latter objective (see "Bibliography"). The thinking analyzed here will follow the precepts in the first half of this book to enable the reader to have insight into the application of theory in everyday practice. I will detail the clinical thinking in each instance, but the reader is advised to consider first, "what do I think in this situation," before proceeding with the author's analysis.

Case #1

Two lines of reasoning merge in the case of the 4-month-old child with fever, shock and coma, as they often do in pediatric practice. First questions include data and hypotheses to examine the homeostatic status of the patient. Paramount in the physician's mind is stabilized life support systems simultaneous with initial attempts to reach a diagnosis. Thus, *homeostatic* and *diagnostic* reasoning occur almost simultaneously.

Data must be utilized both from the patient and from the knowledge of the physician. The patient's data takes the form of specific answers to critical questions and occurs rapidly and calmly.

First, is the child in shock? His initial appearance suggests shock, and thus the first data collected is to answer this question. Simultaneously, the physician asks a quick series of related questions: (1) Is the airway patent? (2) Is the heart stopped? (3) Is circulation impaired in any way? Rapidly the physician determines that (1) the child is breathing without obstruction but at an abnormally low rate, (2) the heart beat is evident at a rapid rate, and (3) the blood pressure is abnormally low. Summary: The child is in shock with respiratory failure but with cardiac function thus far intact. These hypotheses generated are not specific anatomic or etiologic diagnoses but represent explanatory statements of the current status of vital systems. At this point it makes no difference what has produced these homeostatic imbalances, since, if they are not corrected, the patient may die. Elaborate tests are not needed; in fact, they are contraindicated. One does not need pulmonary gas determinations, circulatory rates, or measures of cardiac output to verify the clinical hypotheses—the only "test" is the physical signs of systems failure.

Even as these initial "impressions" are formed and therapeutic steps undertaken, the diagnostic thinking is proceeding. The examiner notes the fever and the hurriedly obtained history of a preceding febrile respiratory illness and begins formulating likely hypotheses, utilizing at first the sequential diagnostic approach which emphasizes probable causes rather than all possibilities. The clinician thinks, "He probably has meningitis, pneumonia or bacteremia." These hypotheses are formulated on the dual grounds of patient data and of medical knowledge. The infant is febrile ("most often means infection"), has historical evidence of a febrile upper respiratory infection ("implies locus of infection which may harbor bacterial pathogens which spread to blood, lungs or meninges"). We know that 4-month-olds experience severe bacterial infections with pneumonia, *Hemophilus influenzae* and meningococci, among a few others. Therefore, we are prepared to meld the specific findings in this infant with the known manifestation of diseases commonly afflicting this age group.

Why does the clinician "select" bacterial causes and initially give scant thought to viral etiology? There are several reasons: (1) There are conditions in which successful therapy is available, (2) certain diagnostic steps will have to occur in sequence, and (3) accurate diagnosis is essential to initiation of therapy. Even if the child has an untreatable cause (e.g., viremia or encephalitis), ultimately one must consider treatable ones in order not to miss them.

As both homeostatic and diagnostic reasoning continue, the clinician begins to apply measures to reverse imbalanced homeostasis. He starts an intravenous line, gives normal saline in calculated amounts, administers oxygen, warms the infant and follows the response with frequent assessment of vital signs, level of response, and recovery of central nervous system (CNS) abnormalities.

In this instance, he is rewarded with prompt return of color, increase in blood pressure, and reestablishment of a normal respiratory pattern.

Attention is then focused on accumulation of more data, first from the physical examination and then by elaboration of history. It is established that the infant is febrile and has a stiff neck and full fontanel. The initial differential now narrows, with bacterial meningitis as the highly probable cause and with viral aseptic meningitis and encephalitis as less likely but possible causes. Although CNS hemorrhage (possibly secondary to trauma) and space-occupying lesions are possible, the presence of fever, nuchal regularity, the preceding febrile upper respiratory infection, and increasing irritability for 2 days all support an acute, infectious process.

The clinician now faces a slight dilemma:

He wishes to test the hypotheses, but in what sequence? A total white blood cell (WBC) count might be done, and blood gases, pH and electrolytes are useful determinants of homeostasis. But the single *best* test is examination of cerebrospinal fluid. It makes no difference what the WBC count will show, a cerebrospinal examination will still be necessary. Therefore, a delay to await WBC results is unnecessary at best and dangerous at worst. Delay in diagnosis and treatment of meningitis could be lethal or result in increased morbidity. Therefore, as soon as the patient is stable a lumbar puncture is performed to establish or refute the major hypotheses. (This child had bacterial meningitis.)

I will not belabor subsequent events, as our focus is on the emergency and thinking surrounding it.

Case #2

With the 2-year-old in Case #2, a single reasonable hypothesis can be established immediately. The combination of history, sudden onset and compatible clinical symptoms and signs points to acute iron poisoning. It is unnecessary initially to consider all causes of vomiting of blood. This may seem to be narrow-minded to some diagnosticians but, in fact, is the only sensible *initial* way to think about the problem. Why?

First, the necessity for a correct specific diagnosis, as well as homeostatic assessment, is evident. Removal of any residual iron, diagnostic serum assessment, and specific therapy will have to be instituted promptly if the diagnosis is correct. Although other causes (hypotheses) are conceivable, they are not probable. Thus, a sequential diagnostic sequence is put into place, with the most likely cause attacked first.

In this child, homeostasis must be assessed and maintained irrespective of specific etiology, but specific measures also must be put into the initial "action." Hence, shock is diagnosed and combated with appropriate measures. At the same time, a dose of ipecac is given in an effort to rid the gastrointestinal tract of further iron and is followed by gastric lavage and bicarbonate instillation (to de-crease absorption of residual iron by conversion of the ferrous form to ferric).

Diagnostic studies are obtained (analysis of emesis specimen and gastric lavage fluid for iron, plus serum iron level), and a decision made on specific chelation. Further discussion of therapy is beyond this chapter, and appropriate texts should be consulted.

Only if the diagnostic tests or the clinical cause belies the diagnosis are further hypotheses generated and tested. The situation presented by this child is quite different from that presented by emesis of blood, with no history of opportunity for, or ingestion of, iron-containing medication, and will be considered in Chapter 17.

The point here is that sequential and specific diagnosis is called for, and restricted thinking is not only allowable but mandatory.

Case #3

The 6-year-old child in Case #3 presents a classic dilemma in emergency pediatric thinking, in contrast to the rather straightforward approach in Case #2. It is the dilemma of antecedents, or a typical chicken-egg analysis. Did the child fall as a result of a CNS event and convulsion, or did the fall result in a CNS event, convulsion and subsequent clinical findings?

In approaching this diagnostic dilemma the physician is also faced with a therapeutic one: Does he simply control the seizure activity and "wait it out," or does he immediately call the neurosurgeon and undertake diagnostic measures to determine if there has been a significant CNS hemorrhage?

First in the line of reasoning is to assess homeostasis; second, to determine extent of injury; and third, to reach a definitive diagnosis. The degree of deviation from normal cognitive function is moderate; therefore, some time is afforded to accomplish other objectives. Had the child been in status epilepticus, with rapidly failing cognitive function, deepening coma and manifest focal signs, no time would have been afforded for pursuit of a leisurely differential diagnosis. Under these circumstances, immediate stabilization and joint medical-neurosurgical evaluation must occur, with the decision to enter the cranial vault hanging in the balance.

This line of reasoning does not mean a lazy pace. Movement from homeostatic evaluation to rapid scan for additional injuries (e.g., broken bones, visceral damage) is immediately followed by specific neurologic assessment.

Neurologic assessment should be designed to test the two extreme hypotheses. First, is a significant intracranial hemorrhage present? Only with reasonable assurance that it either is not, or at least is not rapidly, progressive should assessment of an underlying convulsive disorder be undertaken. Again a form of sequential reasoning, in this case dictated by risk/benefit consideration. If hemorrhage is present, it must be diagnosed and treated. Therefore, despite the differential diagnosis, initial testing involves ruling in, or ruling out, hemorrhage.

The clinician in this instance argues from the patient's standpoint: What is the greatest risk to him? Obviously, the answer is clear, and steps are taken to detect the presence of a subdural or epidural hemorrhage. Immediate neurologic evaluation by a consultant neurosurgeon, noninvasive assessment of intracranial structures (computerized axial tomographic scan), and repeated, frequent neurologic examination searching for changes in the level of consciousness, in vital signs, in the appearance and character of focal signs, and in seizure activity are all undertaken.

Only if all signs are negative and remain stable or diminish does further nonsurgical observation occur with the second hypothesis (i.e., that a convulsive disorder exists and is responsible for the fall and current neurologic signs, e.g., Todd's paralysis and postictal state).

GENERALIZATIONS

These patients and others like them generate a system of emergency thinking that has some generic principles as the guiding force behind it:

1. Homeostatic disturbance is critical to survival, almost without respect to cause. Therefore, *immediate and comprehensive homeostatic assessment is mandatory in all emergencies.*
2. Once homeostatic balance is assured, the diagnostic process is paramount. Thus, *specific etiologic diagnoses must be undertaken simultaneous with, or shortly after, homeostatic assessment and measures to insure stability.*
3. The exact diagnostic approach will vary with the patient, problem and specific circumstances. No one can give a single formula for all. But, *the specific reasoning process will always be found in a risk/benefit analysis on behalf of the patient.*
4. In many emergency situations, *sequential diagnosis is not only allowable but mandatory.*
5. In general, *a complete differential diagnosis* is mandated by high risk to the patient, with specific etiologic diagnoses included which are both diagnosable and treatable.
6. The entire process is usually rapid and occasionally of immediate nature, but it also must be inclusive of pertinent acts and exclusive of unnecessary and time-wasting actions. Thus, *efficiency of diagnosis is critical in emergency thinking.*
7. Diagnosis often necessitates expert consultation. One of the critical elements in emergency care is the *early and correct choice of appropriate expert consultations.*

HOMEOSTATIC DIAGNOSIS

Assessment of homeostasis involves the following elements:

1. Assurance of patent airway
2. Assurance of intact circulation
3. Assurance of respiratory competence
4. Evaluation of fluid and electrolyte balance
5. Assessment of neuromuscular function
6. Nutritional assessment

Rapid analysis of cardiorespiratory integrity involves inspection of the upper airway (nose and pharynx, and supralaryngeal structures in some instances), listening for noise associated with turbulent air flow secondary to obstruction (inspiratory stridor, expiratory wheezing), gauging the adequacy of rate, depth and effectiveness of air flow from the naso-oropharynx to alveoli by both observation and auscultation, consideration of such vital signs as pulse rate, blood pressure and respiratory rate, and palpation, percussion and auscultation of the heart.

Estimation of color, heat and turgor of the skin assist in both cardiorespiratory and fluid balance assessment. Further, the appearance of the eyes (sunken or protruding), the anterior fontanel in infants (distended, flat or depressed), and the subcutaneous tissues (edematous or not) contributes to the overall assessment of the state of hydration. Specific signs of specific anion/cation disturbance are sought (e.g., tetany in Ca^{++} depletion).

Neuromuscular evaluation includes assessment of state of consciousness, response to obvious stimuli, strength, balance and muscular function, specific neurologic signs, such as cranial and peripheral nerve function, and careful examination of all aspects of the eyes.

Nutritional assessment involves overall judgement as to undernutrition, and specific judgement as to presence of single or multiple deficiencies in nutritional components (e.g., vitamin C deficiency with signs of scurvy).

I've detailed some of the features of assessment, not to give a detailed guide but to point out how *little* needs to be done in a short time to gauge the patient's homeostatic status. More elaborate assessment can follow and is often necessary (e.g., to judge the precise degree of hydration or to identify specific electrolyte levels). Often, all that is needed initially is clinical judgement to determine (1) the measures necessary now (e.g., fluid administration in impending shock) and (2) the pace at which the clinician can approach other features of the diagnostic process.

SPECIFIC ETIOLOGIC DIAGNOSIS

To establish a specific etiologic diagnosis the clinician begins by asking two questions: (1) what *most* likely is causing this patient's illness? and (2) what is the entire range of possibilities to explain the process? In some instances, only Question 1 will be addressed; in most, Question 2 will also have to be answered. Several factors dictate the choice between the depth of a single hypothesis versus the breadth of many hypotheses. First and foremost are the specific characteristics of individual patient encounters. The patient with hemoptysis who had an ice pick protruding from his chest is quite different from an individual with the same degree of hemoptysis without obvious antecedent course.

A second factor to be separately considered is the risk to the patient.

A third is in the knowledge of the clinician and the extent of his experience. Those who know little will obviously be limited, and those who know much will be better prepared to make this judgement.

RISK/BENEFIT ANALYSIS

Nowhere else in pediatric practice is the repetitive need for risk/benefit assessment as evident as in crisis situations. How far to go in the reasoning process is totally dependent on degrees of risk and benefit to the individual patient. The major elements of this decision process have been described in Chapter 6. For our purposes here, two of these elements will be further discussed.

Risk to a patient is measurable in answer to two questions: (1) if I fail to consider an hypothesis, will the patient suffer unneeded risk of morbidity and mortality? and (2) if I do expose the patient to diagnostic procedures, is there substantial risk versus the potential benefit? What one is doing is constructing a mental table as follows:

	Risk of missing disease	Risk of diagnostic procedure
Limited diagnosis	High	?
Extensive diagnosis	Low	?

Obviously, in specific circumstances the insertions in this table of high or low risk will vary. A lumbar puncture in suspected bacterial meningitis has low risk compared to the high risk of missing the diagnosis if it is present. On the other hand, a lumbar puncture in undiagnosed, increased intracranial pressure has a high risk of injury if the underlying disease is a supratentorial mass.

For each individual instance, the clinician makes such an assessment based upon his knowledge, the clues in the patient's history and physical examination, and the intrinsic risk of the procedure which, in turn, is partially dependent on the skill of the performer, for some procedures.

SEQUENTIAL VERSUS DIFFERENTIAL DIAGNOSIS

Exploration of sequential and differential

diagnoses has been detailed in Chapter 4. In emergency thinking, the clinician is primarily, if not solely, guided by very specific clinical data. What is sought is expedient arrival at a correct diagnosis with due consideration for sufficient inclusiveness. Risk/benefit thinking helps in the choice. So does the knowledge and experience of the thinker. Above all, one must be prepared to "swing" between the two modes as data are collected, hypotheses reevaluated, and risk/benefit ratios reassessed. Rigid fixation on a single approach irrespective of data is wasteful at best and dangerous at worst.

CONSULTATION

As has been illustrated elsewhere in this text, no single physician can command all skills and knowledge needed by his patients. The trick is to recognize this material limitation and to do something about it. In emergencies the critical issue is to call on the right people at the right time. No dissertation can give specific guidelines for every clinical circumstance. The patient's problem and the specific limitation of the primary physician will determine who is consulted and how quickly.

Emergency consultants are of four types: (1) a more experienced generalist, (2) a specific diagnostician(s), (3) a specific therapeutist, and (4) someone who can supply specific information, such as toxicologic data or appropriate laboratory tests or interpretation thereof.

Since a potent factor in etiologic diagnosis

and risk/benefit judgement is experience, it often is necessary to have a more mature clinician rethink the problem with you. In this way, a more precise definition of the approach to be used and of the actual risks involved becomes possible.

A specific consultant (e.g., a neurologist, a surgeon, etc.) may be useful in interpretation of clinical data as well as in diagnostic analysis. The obvious advantage here is the greater *depth* of knowledge provided.

If a therapeutic maneuver is possible or probable (e.g., bronchoscopy, surgical operation, etc.), the logical time to involve the consultant is early in the diagnostic process. The individual consultant will often function in providing the necessary manual skill. Further, the earliest diagnostic steps taken can be keyed to the future procedure that is contemplated. For example, a blood specimen drawn for culture can be expanded and sent for type and cross match early, if surgery is probable.

Some consultations are very specifically addressed at resolution of a single, or just a few, questions in the overall assessment. One may wish to know the contents of a toxic agent, or the appropriate specimen to submit to microbiology, or the correct roentgenogram to be obtained.

SUMMARY

This chapter has dissected the type of reasoning necessary in emergencies. It considers homeostatic assessment, specific etiologic diagnostic processes and risk/benefit analysis as they apply to an emergent clinical situation.

Chapter 8

Clinical Problem Solving in Febrile Children

INTRODUCTION

The child with fever as a major or sole presenting symptom is one of the commonest problems encountered in pediatrics. The reason for the frequency probably lies in the fact that (1) most febrile illnesses are infectious, (2) the fever results from endogenous pyrogen (EP) release, and (3) infections are common occurrences in infants and children and common antecedents to EP release. Most children have primary experience with a host of pathogens in the first months to years of life; hence, they are not "immune" and react to such onslaught with a brisk and vigorous inflammatory response. One consequence of this infectious immunologic virginity is a massive production of EP, and hence fever.

The child with fever poses specific questions to the physician:

1. Is fever truly present?
2. Is the fever symptomatic of serious disease?
3. Will the fever itself be dangerous to this child?
4. How can I sort out the rare, risky situations from the common, nonthreatening ones?
5. How should I approach the problem of acute fever with few or no focal findings?
6. Apart from the underlying disease, how should I treat the fever itself?
7. In instances of prolonged fever of unknown origin, how do I proceed?

These questions with the accompanying diagnostic reasoning will be addressed in this chapter.

THE GENESIS OF FEVER

To understand better the specific diagnostic and therapeutic approach to fever, we must have some grasp of why fever occurs and its dangers and benefits. Temperature control is vested in hypothalamic function, with sensory and regulatory mechanisms housed in the preoptic area. The "thermostat" is usually set in a narrow range, for most persons at 37 ± 0.5 to $0.7°C$. Maintenance of steady body temperatures is dependent upon perception, in the hypothalamus and skin, of tissue temperature; and minor adjustments in heat loss and heat gain mechanisms are signaled by the hypothalamus.

Fever usually results from a change in the "thermostat" setting to a higher level, falsely leading the hypothalamic receptors to believe that the body is "cool" (in comparison to the setting). Heat gain mechanisms are set into motion, such as shivering, agitation, hunger and increased metabolic activity. Simultaneously, heat loss is conserved by vasoconstriction, erection of hair, and attempts to decrease surface area for radiation loss reduction (curling up). Hence, the typical result is a flushed, shivering, irritable child who pulls his arms and legs onto his abdomen and chest and burrows into the bedcovers.

Why is the thermostat setting altered? The alteration almost always results from circulating EP which is a small protein or group of proteins. EP is produced by many cells (phagocytes, monocytes, macrophages, and reticuloendothelial system cells) in response to infectious agents, antitoxin, pyrogenic steroids, and antigen-antibody complexes and by phagocytosis itself.

Fever also occurs as a result of restrictive heat loss (e.g., sunstroke) or excessive heat gain (e.g., hypermetabolic states) in which imbalance between production and loss occurs.

This brief physiologic excursion helps us in recognizing that (1) fever often is a response to infection or inflammation through increase in EP, 2) symptoms are attributable to fever itself and need not be linked with other disease, and (3) the therapeutic approach often is directly aimed at resetting the thermostat and indirectly aimed at eliminating the stimulus for EP production or altering the gain/loss ratio.

THE MAJOR PROBLEMS POSED BY FEVER

Ordinarily, the first task facing the clinician is to determine whether fever is truly present. In many individuals the fluctuation of body temperature is a diurnal event, and alterations of 1° from "normal" are simply manifestations of statistical distribution of normality and not of underlying disease. Certainly, despite the simplicity of obtaining body temperatures, many unsophisticated parents have no real knowledge of how to take and record body temperatures accurately. Anecdotal reports of individual physicians are backed by several studies which illustrate the need to ascertain that the body temperature was, in fact, accurately assessed. Such simple procedures as not returning a mercury thermometer from a previous high setting to below normal prior to obtaining a temperature often complicates interpretation.

A second component of determination of fever's presence is the rare, but difficult, situation in which fever is factitiously produced either by the patient or parent. Usually the child or parents have psychologic reasons for wishing to report the presence of fever, and hence disease, which discussion is beyond the scope of this chapter. In cases of sustained high fever without any obvious cause, and with a well-appearing child, the physician is advised to record the temperature personally or have it recorded by an objective third party, such as a nurse or other health personnel. The entire procedure of temperature taking must be accomplished by the objective observer from entering the room until the temperature is actually recorded from the thermometer. At no point during this process should the patient or parents be left alone. If factitious fever is diagnosed, the problem of the psychological reasons must be addressed directly, although it is beyond the scope of this chapter. Under no circumstances should factitious fever be treated as a trivial event, as it often signals a very disturbed emotional relationship.

Assuming fever is present, the physician must gauge its extent and the presence of other symptoms or signs which are suggestive of the underlying cause. In many infants and children, fever of substantial proportion readily occurs even with minor infectious insults. In fact, each individual appears to have a febrile response pattern peculiar to himself, and the experienced clinician will learn with time how each patient responds. Thus, one infant who develops temperatures in excess of 104° to 105° with each minor respiratory infection is viewed differently from the child who never generates much fever with minor infections and now presents with a very high temperature.

Many infants and children will have fever with relatively little in the way of objective signs or symptoms. This is particularly true if the parents bring the patient to the physician's attention very early in the course of an illness. If, after a diligent physical examination, no signs are uncovered, the physician's course should usually be one of watchful waiting. Administration of liberal fluid intake, with or without antipyretics, is often selected during the watchful waiting period. The use of antibiotics should not be overdone. They may mask subsequent elevations of body temperature or reduce specific symptoms, especially pain, which may lead the physician to the correct diagnosis. As a general rule, fever which produces little or only moderate symptomatology in the infant or child should not be treated vigorously during the observational period. However, once it is determined that a serious infection or process is not present, temperature relief often reduces patient discomfort.

Moderate temperature elevations are of no consequence to most patients. Unless the patient has a severe underlying disease in which fever itself may produce adverse consequences, there is usually no serious consequence of the temperature elevation. Despite teleologic reasoning that suggests fever would not be present unless it had some benefit, there is little objective evidence to indicate that fever itself is beneficial to the host. Claims have been made that it improves the host defense mechanisms, creates an environment antagonistic to an infectious organism's growth, and assists in slowing down the patient at a time when all of his energy should be mustered toward the resolution of the inflammatory process. None of these claims have been followed by objective evidence that any of these mechanisms are, in fact, true in the intact host.

Rapidly rising body temperatures and high sustained temperatures do pose a risk to some children. In a few percent of any given population, rapidly increasing fever will be accompanied by febrile convulsion. Usually this is a single episode without sustained convulsive activity. Experts have argued for years whether the single episode in itself is dangerous to the child and whether or not it heralds an underlying convulsive disorder. As of this writing, there is no clear resolution to this dilemma, and most experts now recommend a very conservative approach to the management of an initial febrile convulsion and to subsequent anticonvulsant prophylaxis. Again, this is beyond the scope of this chapter.

Very high fevers that occasionally occur when the temperature regulation mechanism is completely destroyed, either by environmental causes, such as excessive exposure to heat, or by ingestion of certain toxins, such as lead, do pose a hazard to the patient. Extensive cerebral damage, and even death, may result in such circumstances. Vigorous measures to control body temperature and to treat the underlying cause should be employed in such circumstances.

Most commonly, the physician confronted with a febrile child must decide whether a relatively trivial cause, such as a viral upper respiratory tract infection, is present, or a more significant, more treatable etiology is responsible for fever. No textbook can summarize all the individual situations that the clinician can encounter, and a carefully performed history and physical examination are the only guides to accurate diagnosis. In the presence of focal signs the clinician must decide whether the extent of fever is accounted for by the focal infection. Thus a febrile child who has a bulging, erythematous tympanic membrane most likely has otitis media as a cause of his fever. Among hundreds and hundreds of such children there will be an occasional child whose infection will have spread beyond the focal site and invaded either the bloodstream or distant organs. In many such circumstances, physical examination will give a clue to the presence of distant infection in such sites as the meninges.

Occasionally it will be impossible to determine from physical examination alone that a given infant has, in fact, disseminated his focal infection. Thus, the clinician must constantly be alert for a cluster of signs, the presence of which will signal him to undertake further diagnostic tests. For example, in a child with bilateral otitis media and fever, the degree and quality of the inevitable irritability that is present must be gauged accurately. If the irritability occurs when the child's ears are manipulated, or during the physical examination, but he becomes totally consolable when held in the parent's arms, the physician may be tempted to treat only the otitis media without pursuing further studies. On the other hand, if the child's irritability is manifest throughout the observational period, irrespective of whether he is consoled or not, this most often is an indication for exploring the possibility that bacterial meningitis is present. Again, one cannot anticipate every single clinical combination that will occur in actual practice. The most important lesson to be learned here is that following a thorough history and physical examination, observation of the infant may be critical to subsequent determinations. Risk/benefit reasoning and the principle of commonness, discussed earlier, often dictate the physician's approach. If in summing up the clinical situation the clinician decides that the risk of not diagnosing meningitis is greater than the risk of the procedures to be employed, he will perform a lumbar puncture. Similarly, if the clinician has absolutely no reason to suspect other than otitis media, he will permit the law of commonness to dictate his subsequent action in treating the child solely for otitis media while arranging careful follow-up.

Acute fever which is unaccompanied by any focal finding for several days poses a special circumstance in evaluation. We know that a number of viral infections, including roseola and some of the enteroviral illnesses, will produce fever with no other clinical features. We also know that some infections remain hidden from even a careful historian and examiner (e.g., urinary tract infections). Further, it is clear that many individuals with noninfectious disease may initially present with temperature elevations and no other physical findings. This knowledge leads us to a unified approach to the febrile child without clinical manifestations. First, the child should not be treated blindly with either antipyretic or antimicrobial therapy. To do so runs the risk of masking significant clinical findings that may develop as the child's illness progresses. Most cases of missed bacterial meningitis occur in a setting in which a febrile child was treated with antimicrobial agents without real cause. The clinician is then chagrined to discover, hours or days later, that in reality the child had bacterial meningitis, and that he (the clinician) has managed to suppress symptoms without curing the disease.

Second, continued observation and close, careful follow-up with reexamination as indicated will help to clarify most of these problems with time. If, on initial presentation, the child does not appear ill despite the temperature elevation, the clinician's wisest course is simply to do nothing. By doing nothing we do not imply neglect or discharge of the patient, but rather careful instructions to the parent as to what to anticipate in the way of positive findings that may occur, and telephonic communication in both directions

during the course of the child's febrile illness. Further, if the fever is sustained for several days, reexamination of the child at intervals is desirable. In a few instances, to be discussed more fully later, the early stages of noninfectious diseases, such as rheumatoid arthritis, may present with fever and little else. Only continued observation in these circumstances will heighten the clinician's suspicion that a noninfectious cause is present.

"Hidden" infections pose a special problem. Most often, there is no direct way, particularly in infants, to suspect the presence of such infections as those of the urinary tract. Given an infant or child with fever and no other complaints, some clinicians prefer to use so-called screening tests to help guide their future diagnostic probes. The most commonly employed is the total white blood cell count and differential. Provided the clinician recognizes the limitations of this procedure, its judicious use is warranted. Extreme changes in the white blood cell count (i.e., very high counts or very low counts or marked disturbances in the proportion of polymorphonuclear leukocytes and lymphocytes) may give a direct clue to the type of infection in the individual and dictate further diagnostic tests, such as blood culture, lumbar puncture, or search for specific viruses.

On the other hand, an undistinguished total white blood cell count or differential does not rule out the presence of any of the more serious infections that the clinician is considering. In essence, a normal white cell count simply reemphasizes the need for continued observation as above. Other clinicians employ the so-called acute phase reactants. Among these are the erythrocyte sedimentation rate, the C-reactive protein, and the platelet count. The use of these tests, either singly or in combination, does not appear to enhance significantly the clinician's observation or the clinician's observation coupled with the white cell count. *In most acute febrile situations, they are unnecessary and wasteful.* Further, they do not substitute for continued observation and reperformed physical examinations as indicated.

On the other hand, the urinalysis is an underused technique in acutely febrile children, particularly infants. Urinary tract infections may be suspected by examination of urinary sediment through a variety of techniques. What is sought is a specimen representing bladder urine that avoids urethral or skin contamination. In older children a midstream urine specimen, and in young infants a suprapubic aspiration, will provide such a specimen. The presence of white blood cells and/or bacteria is reason enough to suspect a urinary tract infection and demand that the specimen be cultured and, if positive, the child be treated and subsequently examined for urinary tract anomalies.

PROLONGED FEVER OF UNKNOWN ORIGIN (PFUO)

In adults a fever is not considered prolonged unless 2 weeks have elapsed since onset and no obvious cause has been determined, including a period of observation in the hospital. These criteria have been applied to children but to most pediatricians appear too stringent. We begin to become concerned if a child has had fever for longer than 4 or 5 days without obvious cause. The reason for the difference is that most causes of acute fever in children will become manifest in a very short period of time, if they are to be manifest at all. Thus, as the interval prolongs beyond 3 or 4 days we must begin to suspect origins of fever other than the usual causes.

A number of studies have been conducted looking at groups of children with PFUO. Most studies show basically the same proportion and types of disease. By far the largest group, comprising 40 to 50% of all such children, is infectious causes. They range from occult urinary tract infections to infections of the bone, central nervous system and other organs of the body. The second largest category is collagen vascular disease, the most prominent of which is juvenile rheumatoid arthritis (JRA). In children, particularly in young children and infants, a common form of presentation for JRA is prolonged fever with little or no joint manifestations. Occasionally the infant may be irritable when limbs are moved, suggesting arthralgia, although objective signs of arthritis are seldom present.

A third category, comprising a smaller percentage of the total, is malignant disease. Lymphomas, leukemia, and solid tumors are included in this category. In each series, then, there is a scattering of individual causes occurring in fewer than 1% of instances and involving extremely rare diseases of metabolic, central nervous system or other origin. Table 8.1 summarizes the common causes in several series reported in the literature.

Diagnostic and Therapeutic Suggestions

From all of this experience, coupled with the author's own, a series of diagnostic and therapeutic suggestions has emerged.

1. Viral infections are more often the cause of PFUO in children than adults.

2. Among upper respiratory infections, otitis media and sinusitis were frequently "hidden" causes of PFUO.

3. Streptococcosis associated with minimal upper respiratory tract signs and symptoms can occur in young infants. It is due to Group A streptococcal infections in the immunologic virgin.

4. Pneumonia of varying etiology, including tuberculous and fungal, must be considered.

5. The urinary tract, central nervous system, bones and bloodstream may all be infected in infants and children, with PFUO as the only overt manifestation.

6. Infectious mononucleosis is occasionally difficult to diagnose in young children and can present as a prolonged fever of unknown origin. Diligent search for the presence of a spleen, the presence of a rash, or other focal signs may aid in suggesting this diagnosis.

7. Specific rare infections, such as brucellosis, malaria, typhus, and cat-scratch fever, occur with an unpredictable pattern and rarely. Thus, they may be extremely difficult to diagnose unless appropriate epidemiologic clues are provided in the history.

8. Infections of bone occasionally will offer little in the way of specific localizing signs. One symptom to be wary of is pseudoparalysis in which an infant fails to move a single limb, or moves it with difficulty, suggesting a neurologic cause when, in fact, underlying bone pain produces the immobility.

Table 8.1
Children with PFUO—Series Reported Since 1965 Related to Ultimate Diagnoses

Date:	1965	1972	1975	1977
Author:	Brewis*	McClung†	Pizzo‡	Lohr§
Locale:	Newcastle, England	Madison, WI	Boston, MA	Charlottesville, VA
Setting:	General practice	Childrens Hospital	Childrens Hospital	University Hospital
No. of patients:	165	99	100	54
Age range:	"Children"	0–16 yr	0–14+ yr	5 mo–14 yr
Infection:	91 (55%)	29 (29%)	52 (52%)	18 (33%)
URI‖	30	7	10	2
LRI	24	8	4	
UTI	10	4	4	3
GI	8	1	2	1
Bone	2	0	2	1
CNS	0	4	3	3
Blood	0	0	2	0
SBE	0	1	3	1
Abscess	5	0	0	1
Brucella	2	1	0	0
Tbc	5	2	1	3
Mononucleosis	5	1	2	1
Viral	0	0	18	2
Malaria	0	0	1	0
Collagen vascular	9 (5)	11 (12)	20 (20)	11 (20)
Neoplasms	3 (2)	8 (8)	6 (6)	7 (13)
Other (+)	18 (10)	19 (19)	10 (10)	8 (15)
Unknown	44 (28)	32 (32)	12 (12)	10 (19)

* Brewis, EG: Undiagnosed fever. *Br Med J* 1:107, 1965.
† McClung, HJ: Prolonged fever of unknown origin in children. *JAMA* 124:544, 1972.
‡ Pizzo, PA, Lovejoy, FH, and Smith, DH: Prolonged fever in children: Review of 100 cases. *Pediatrics* 55:468, 1975.
§ Lohr, JA, and Hendley, JO: Prolonged fever of unknown origin, a record of experiences with 54 childhood patients. *Clin Pediat* 16:768, 1977.
‖ Abbreviations: URI, upper respiratory infection; LRI, lower respiratory infection; UTI, urinary tract infection; GI, gastrointestinal; CNS, central nervous system; SBE, subacute bacterial endocarditis; Tbc, tuberculosis.

9. Tuberculosis should be considered in many infants with prolonged fever of unknown origin in which other causes have been ruled out.

10. JRA and regional enteritis commonly masquerade as PFUO. Other forms of noninfectious inflammatory disease are much less common and, unless there are specific signs pointing to multisystem involvement, may be difficult to diagnose. Frequently, only continued observation accompanied by nonspecific laboratory tests (to be discussed below) yields such diagnoses.

11. Among infrequent causes are various congenital and metabolic syndromes, including lesions near or in the hypothalamus, diabetes insipidus, and various ectodermal dysplasias.

12. Surprisingly, immunodeficiency is seldom a cause of PFUO. Most commonly, children with immunodeficiencies have abundant clinical manifestations of their infectious processes.

13. In a child who is being administered therapy, particularly antibiotics, drug fever often presents as PFUO. This diagnosis may

be extremely difficult except by excluding other causes and eliminating the drug in question.

14. Factitious fever occurs rarely in all series and must be considered as discussed previously.

Clues to Diagnosis of PFUO

It is also clear from consideration of multiple cases of PFUO that there are some helpful and some nonhelpful clues as to underlying diagnosis.

1. The pattern of fever is not helpful in most situations. Only in malaria does the pattern of fever suggest the specific underlying cause.

2. The duration of fever is also not helpful.

3. The degree of illness or "toxicity" associated with fever is not helpful.

4. The response to antipyretics does not help in most instances. Some individuals feel that JRA is an exception to this generalization in that a therapeutic trial with aspirin, after all other causes have been excluded, may result in a cessation of fever and that removal of aspirin some weeks later may result in a recurrence of the pattern, suggesting but not proving that JRA is present.

5. Response to antibiotics is not specifically helpful. As indicated previously, this often is a two-edged sword in which serious underlying bacterial disease is manifest but not halted. However, in some situations, the blind use of antibiotics with a response often leads the clinician to an intensive search for underlying infectious cause after antibiotics have been removed. This course is not recommended, in that the same search may be suggested if more time were given to the observational period.

6. Abdominal pain is not a discriminatory finding in most instances. Many children will have this symptom without reference to intra-abdominal disease. However, should abdominal pain occur consistently in conjunction with PFUO, such diseases as regional enteritis should be considered in the differential diagnosis.

7. Nonspecific central nervous system symptoms often do not indicate underlying central nervous system disease. Headache, dizziness, vomiting, eye pain—all can occur in the absence of central nervous system lesions.

8. When a skin rash occurs in a child with PFUO, one must consider collagen vascular disease or malignancy. The nature of the rash often will assist in this differential.

9. In patients with collagen vascular disease, musculoskeletal symptoms are prominent, even if specific signs of arthritis are absent.

10. The presence of lymphadenopathy does not help to discriminate among the various infectious or noninfectious causes.

11. The presence of severe respiratory findings, such as cyanosis or dyspnea, often correlates with potentially lethal disease. The presence of these findings in a patient with PFUO should result in an urgent search for underlying cardiovascular and pulmonary diseases. Bacterial endocarditis particularly must be ruled out in such circumstances.

12. Murmurs are often nondiagnostic, in that hemic sounds are produced with the high flow that accompanies febrile states. However, in some instances of endocarditis the presence of a murmur may be specifically suggestive of this diagnosis.

13. Hepatosplenomegaly is seldom a useful differential finding. It occurs nonspecifically in so many causes of PFUO due to reticulo-endothelial hyperplasia that it does not often point in a single direction.

The laboratory approach to the diagnosis of PFUO should follow the hypotheses that can be set, given all the previous considerations. We know that, most frequently, infectious or noninfectious inflammatory disease will be present. Thus, our search is aimed in both directions simultaneously and sequentially. Initially, nonspecific diagnostic aids are coupled with specific diagnostic probes, looking for the presence of infection and, simultaneously, for the indirect evidence of a noninfectious inflammatory process.

The total white blood cell count is often not useful. However, the presence in the differential of increased numbers of polymorphonuclear leukocytes may occur in collagen vascular disease as well as in bacterial infections. Occasionally, viral infections will also masquerade with an increased polymorphonuclear count, reducing the differential diagnostic value of this finding.

Lymphoblasts should be sought in peripheral smears in leukemia, even though they are not present in a fair percentage at the onset of the disease.

Anemia is common but does not discriminate among the many causes.

In contrast to the situation in acute febrile states, an elevated erythrocyte sedimentation rate may be useful in suspecting collagen vascular disease, malignancy, and chronic infectious diseases, such as tuberculosis. The presence of persistently elevated erythrocyte sedimentation rate in a patient with PFUO should intensify the search in these areas.

The urinalysis is infrequently abnormal, but may provide valuable clues in specific patients to the presence of urinary tract infection or endocarditis.

In collagen vascular disease, alterations in the albumin/globulin ratio and disturbances in the alpha and beta globulins are frequently observed. Occasionally, a hyperimmunoglobulinemia may occur in collagen vascular disease or in chronic infection. Rarely, a specific immunoglobulin deficiency may be detected in a patient with PFUO.

Chest radiographs are occasionally useful, since they are positive in some instances with no clinical clues to specific chest disease, especially in such diseases as tuberculosis. When specific clinical clues are present, suggesting such disease, the chest radiogram often has a high yield. Regional radiography is useful when one is considering urinary tract infections, inflammatory disease of the gastrointestinal tract, and bone infections or malignancies. The use of the various types of scans has probably been overdone as these new techniques have been introduced. Encouraging reports occur as each new scanning device is introduced, but with their application across this broad group of patients their usefulness generally diminishes. False positives and false negatives have both occurred in patients with PFUO, and reliance on the various scans to provide a magical diagnosis is senseless.

In many instances a specific search for infectious disease can be instituted by repetitive blood cultures, examination of the bone marrow both histologically and by culture, and sampling of various sites in which abnormalities are detected (e.g., lung aspiration).

Finally, judicious use of biopsies of such organs as the lung, liver and bone marrow may establish specific neoplastic and infectious disease causes of PFUO. In most series, about 40% of biopsies are diagnostic or suggestive of the correct underlying process.

In summary, the approach to the patient with PFUO should include four stages.

1. A detailed history should be taken looking for specific focal symptoms and epidemiologic clues as to environmental contacts that may involve unusual infectious agents. Further, the history should emphasize questions designed to detect undiagnosed but preexistent underlying disease.

2. A detailed and comprehensive physical examination should be performed at the outset and repeated as frequently as is necessary as the PFUO state continues. What is being sought is the presence of focal signs that may lead the clinician to specific diagnostic tests, such as bacterial cultures, viral cultures, or biopsy.

3. The white blood count differential, erythrocyte sedimentation rate and protein analysis offer a reasonable screening panel initially and may be followed up if abnormalities are detected. One must remember the limitations of these procedures and their nonspecific nature. Finally, in some patients, judicious use of radionuclide and computerized axial tomographic scans may reveal focal areas of infection, inflammation or malignancy that are unsuspected from clinical manifestations. However, the random use of these techniques, or their application to every patient with PFUO, may result in false positive or false negative findings which will lead the clinician astray.

4. Often, continued observation is the most valuable diagnostic test. Reiteration of history, repetitive physical examination, and continued surveillance of vital signs, activity, appetite, etc. may yield valuable clues as to the progression of the process and its localization.

Chapter 9

Coma

INTRODUCTION

Coma is defined as the absence of all reflex activity and psychologic responses in an infant or child. Alternatively, the patient may have more moderate coma, with preservation only of primitive reflex motor responses.

The comatose child presents immediate dilemmas to the physician. Simultaneously, diagnostic and therapeutic reasoning must occur along with homeostatic assessment and institution of measures to preserve life and homeostatic balance.

This chapter will explore the clinical reasoning in assessment and management of the comatose state in infants and children. I will proceed by presenting four case histories as examples which we may use to dissect and analyze clinical reasoning.

CASE HISTORIES

Case #1

A 6-month-old infant presents with 3 days of fever, irritability and deepening lethargy. Today the infant failed to be aroused by his parents and was rushed into the emergency room.

A rapid physical assessment reveals the infant to be unresponsive to auditory, visual, and pain stimuli, to lack deep tendon and superficial abdominal reflexes, and to be limp with no active or passive resistance to limb manipulation. The infant has a slightly tense fontanel and supple neck, and the rest of the physical examination is within normal limits.

Vital signs initially are: temperature, 36° C; blood pressure, 90/50; pulse rate, 110/min; and respiratory rate, 20/min. There is no gross physical evidence of trauma, petechiae, purpura or hemorrhage in the skin or subcutaneous tissues. Pupillary reflexes are present but very sluggish, and the doll's eye phenomenon is elicitable.

Case #2

A 6-year-old male is admitted with failure to respond to auditory and painful stimuli. He was well until 1 week ago, when he complained of fatigue, headache and anorexia. These were mild at first, but increased in severity progressively until the present. This afternoon he complained of increasing headache and appeared to go to sleep but was found to be unarousable 1 hour later. When found, he had lost both bowel and bladder control.

Examination revealed a severely obtunded, nonresponsive boy whose deep tendon reflexes were barely elicitable bilaterally. His corneal and pupillary reflexes were present, but his eyes had a roving gaze. No active motion was observed, and minimal passive resistance to limb motion was detected. His vital signs were: temperature, 38.5° C; blood pressure, 160/95; pulse rate, 140/min; and respiratory rate, 16/min.

Case #3

A 15-year-old is brought to the emergency room in a dazed, confused state following collision of his bicycle with a moving automobile. On initial examination he has a blood pressure of 105/70, a pulse rate of 116/min, a respiratory rate of 40/min, and a temperature of 36° C. Bruises and lacerations are present on the left face, scalp, lower arm and the entire lateral surface of his left leg. There is a single large bruise over the lower left chest beginning in the midaxillary line and extending superiorly and anteriorly to the left nipple. The remainder of his examination is negative except for confusion as to person, place or time. He seems to be barely able to follow the examiner's instructions, and he lapses into unresponsiveness with his eyes closed if left alone.

Within the first 20 minutes of assessment he becomes nonarousable by auditory or visual stimuli, and only grimaces slightly when severe painful stimuli are applied. Progressive loss of corneal, pupillary, superficial skin and deep tendon reflexes are observed. His left pupil begins to dilate and remains unresponsive to light. His extremities become rigid, and he assumes a stiff posture with moderate arching of his back, internal rotation of his arms, and clenching of his fingers over his thumbs bilaterally.

Case #4

A 10-year-old female who has been ill with vague complaints of abdominal pain, lethargy, inattentiveness and dysuria for more than 1 week is brought to your office. Her parents and teachers thought she was attempting to avoid school and urged her to attend despite her complaints.

She was discovered slumped on her desk today, the parents were alerted, and she was taken into the emergency room because of her bizarre behavior. By the time the parents arrived, she had become combative, began cursing and speaking to persons not present, and also performed repetitive, nonsensical actions. She finally collapsed on the way to the hospital and became unresponsive.

Her examination revealed an unresponsive girl, with a blood pressure of 90/40, a pulse

rate of 170/min, a respiratory rate of 35/min, and a temperature of 35.6° C.

Her respirations were deep and unlabored, although rapid. She appeared oblivious to all but the most painful stimuli.

On questioning, the parents added only that her dysuria was intermittent, but that she did get up each night to urinate, which was unusual for her. She had also complained of intermittent midabdominal pain throughout the week. The parents vigorously indicated that her bizarre behavior was distinctly unusual for this child.

GENERAL COMMENTS

These four children represent similar final stages of different pathophysiologic processes. Their mental obtundation and loss of all but primitive reflex activity place them into the deep coma state. Coma has been staged by various observers in order to give priority to the urgency of the physician's response and to offer some prognostic insight to the ultimate outcome. In children there is sufficient variation in outcome related to the "stage" of coma as to urge extreme caution in prognostication. On the other hand, the degree of coma and the rate at which it progresses through the various stages are useful as guides to our thinking and to the speed of response.

A commonly used staging is that developed for Reye's syndrome (encephalopathy, and fatty infiltration of the liver of uncertain cause, although occasionally following varicella, influenza-B and other infections):

Stage 1—the patient exhibits lethargy and sleepiness, and the electroencephalogram (EEG) reveals rhythmic slowing with prominent beta waves and rare delta waves.
Stage 2—the patient is disoriented, is often delirious, and becomes combative. The EEG is dysrhythmic, with slow dominant delta waves mixed with some beta waves.
Stage 3—the patient becomes obtunded, comatose, and demonstrates decorticate rigidity with preserved pupillary and doll's eye reflexes. The EEG is identical to that in Stage 2.
Stage 4—the patient displays deepening unresponsiveness, decerebrate rigidity and loss of all reflexes. The EEG becomes disorganized in rhythm with delta waves of low

voltage and brief bursts of isoelectric intervals or suppression.

Stage 5—the patient develops generalized seizures with complete loss of reflexes and respiratory arrest, and the EEG becomes isoelectric or flat.

SPECIFIC CASE ANALYSIS

Case #1

The 6-month-old child in Case #1 offers several clues to the initial clinician. First, his central nervous system manifestations have come about progressively and over a relatively long interval. This suggests a continuous process that had its origin in the early manifestations. Since these were fever and irritability, one immediately suspects an infection of the central nervous system. Thus, given the history alone, the clinician already establishes one working hypothesis that will be strengthened or weakened as he progresses through the physical examination.

Stage 1 coma appears to be present in this infant, although an EEG will not be performed. The presence of fever and the slightly tense fontanel immediately confirm in the clinician's mind his initial impression of a primary central nervous system process. Since the child is 6 months old, the most likely central nervous system lesion is meningitis, either bacterial or viral in nature. Since a risk/benefit analysis indicates that bacterial meningitis must be ruled out, the clinician rapidly proceeds from a generalized hypothesis to several specific etiologic ones to the immediate diagnostic test.

The clinician performs a lumbar puncture which reveals a cloudy fluid (which has 3,900 cells, most of which are polys), a low cerebrospinal fluid glucose, and a normal protein. At this point he need not go further in his diagnostic reasoning, as he has established probable bacterial meningitis as the working hypothesis, which demands immediate therapeutic intervention both to specifically counteract the anticipated bacterial spectrum that may produce this disease and to control increased intracranial pressure. This chapter is not intended to be a lecture on bacterial meningitis, and hence we will end the discussion here. However, the child did have *He-*

mophilus influenzae bacterial meningitis and was successfully treated with chloramphenicol intravenously and restriction of fluid intake until the increased intracranial pressure was controlled.

This child illustrates several principles in the management of coma. First, a rapid clinical assessment indicated to the clinician that he was dealing with a progressive disease which had reached rather minimal stages of coma. He combined a positive physical finding with a history suggestive of central nervous system disease and quickly established a workable hypothesis which could be rapidly tested. Had the spinal fluid been clear, he then could have proceeded to other considerations. However, the most urgent and, from the risk/benefit standpoint, most important disease to rule out in this child was bacterial meningitis. As a result, the clinician applied the definitive test, an examination of cerebrospinal fluid, rather than develop an elaborate differential diagnosis and test each of the hypotheses that could have been formulated. This is an example of sequential diagnostic reasoning discussed in an earlier chapter, which in this case yielded the correct diagnosis with maximum efficiency at minimum cost to the patient.

It is important to remember that the clinician could have been wrong. The child may have had another cause for his coma superimposed on a 3-day illness. However, this sequence is unlikely, and applying the concepts of simplicity and single diagnostic processes, especially in a 6-month-old infant, allows the clinician to function efficiently and smoothly in reaching a correct diagnosis.

It is also possible that the slightly tense fontanel was, in fact, normal, and the clinician may have been misled into overemphasizing a physical finding based on establishing a working hypothesis, into which he was then trying to "fit" the physical findings. This illustrates the absolute need to be as objective as possible in obtaining the best possible data. Even if the tension in the fontanel had been equivocal, the clinician still would have had to consider his primary hypothesis on the risk/benefit basis. Exploration of other causes must take second place to establishing the presence or absence of bacterial meningitis.

A further point illustrated by the diagnostic reasoning in this child is the importance of the physician's knowledge of epidemiology, age-related incidence of disease, and specific knowledge as to the presentation of specific diseases. Despite the fact that we focus in this text on the process of clinical problem solving, it cannot be emphasized with enough clarity and enough emphasis that factual knowledge underlies the process. The best problem solver is also usually the most knowledgeable. However, the most knowledgeable individual may not be the best problem solver. In this child's illness it is essential that the clinician know the major causes of coma at this particular age interval, that he knows the sequence in bacterial meningitis, that he recognizes the primacy of lumbar puncture in establishing the diagnosis, and that he knows the ordinary organisms that produce the disease and their antimicrobial spectrum in order that he might apply correct, immediate therapy. Although he must be be able to string these facts together in a logical sequential series of steps, nevertheless he must have the knowledge in order to do so.

Case #2

In Case #2 we encounter the comatose state in an age group in which it is infrequent. Its onset in this 6-year-old boy is quite different from that of the child in the first case and consists of rather vague findings that are not necessarily localized to any process. The one notable complaint, that of increasing headache, might lead the clinician to consider intracranial causes, inasmuch as this is an uncommon complaint in most prepubertal children. Apart from the manifestations of coma in the physical examination, the striking findings are a relatively normal temperature and a blood pressure that is greatly elevated for his age. The pulse rate is also increased, but the respiratory rate is normal. The clinician links together the onset of headache of increasing severity and the presence of coma, hypertension and tachypnea to suspect that the origin of the central nervous system symptoms relates to some cerebral process. At this point he can formulate his initial hypothesis, that of hypertensive encephalopathy, as a primary working diagnosis

and then consider other intracranial causes, such as intracranial bleeding, which might elevate the blood pressure secondary to stimulation of the appropriate centers.

Also useful in the history is the statement that the child had lost bowel and bladder control. This is strongly suggestive of the patient having experienced a convulsion. The clinician can add to his thinking the fact that hypertensive encephalopathy is probable, since this is a common way in which this disease expresses itself.

The most common cause of acute hypertensive crises in children is of renal origin. Acute glomerulonephritis, pyelonephritis and a variety of other acquired and congenital disorders may lead to hypertension and acute hypertensive encephalopathy. Thus, a highly probable set of circumstances is established in hypothesis setting in this patient. The clinician recognizes that hypertension of renal origin is the single most common cause of the sequence observed and would begin to focus on this diagnosis simultaneously with the homeostatic therapy of controlling the hypertension to prevent further cerebral damage.

As he begins to treat the hypertension the clinician must also consider the possibility that other diseases are producing this child's clinical state. Cardiovascular disorders, such as coarctation of the aorta, must be kept in mind, and a variety of poisonings, infectious disorders and congenital defects must also be kept in mind. In this case the clinician felt it essential to distinguish between disorders of renal origin and intrinsic central nervous system diseases. He ascertained on physical examination that papilledema was not present, retinal hemorrhages were not observed, and focal neurologic signs could not be detected. These negative findings coupled with the history of the slowly progressive disease over the last week suggest that both acute glomerulonephritis with hypertensive encephalopathy and acute encephalitis are the leading considerations. All of the other disorders mentioned above will be sequentially considered if the initial probes fail to establish the most probable causes.

Although we will not discuss this aspect further, it is essential to recognize that concomitant emergency therapy to restore homeostasis (i.e., return blood pressure towards a more normal level) is essential and will run parallel to the diagnostic thinking.

The clinician will reexamine the history to look for signs of streptococcal infection in the few weeks preceding the onset of symptoms, to ascertain whether urinary changes were observed suggestive of hematuria, and to ascertain whether or not any chronic urinary tract symptoms were present or whether episodes suggestive of acute pyelonephritis had occurred in the past. He also will reexamine the patient more carefully for the presence of subtle edema, congestive heart failure and differential blood pressures between the upper and lower limbs. Thus, in very rapid fashion, additional historical and physical examination data help to focus attention on one or the other of the primary diagnoses at the same time that initial testing of the hypotheses is being carried out.

The critical elements in establishing the differential diagnosis from the laboratory standpoint are examination of the urine and the character of the cerebrospinal fluid. Depending on the results of these initial probes, additional renal studies or central nervous system studies may be indicated, but they are not mandated as part of the primary diagnostic process. Thus, antistreptolysin-O titers, complement levels, protein determination and determination of blood urea nitrogen and creatinine in the blood may follow the discovery of microscopic hematuria and proteinuria but would not ordinarily be attempted without this positive urinary finding. Similarly, EEGs and other studies of the central nervous system would not be carried out unless all historical, physical examination and laboratory data were negative in respect to renal disease and cardiovascular disease.

Alternatively, one would be positively directed toward central nervous system diagnostic studies if the spinal fluid were characteristic of encephalitis or meningitis. Thus one can see unfolding the diagnostic reasoning in this comatose child that focuses on renal and central nervous system causes initially and considers other reasons that assist in directing further historical and physical examination probes.

In this particular instance it was discovered that the child did have impetigo 2 weeks prior to the onset of these symptoms and had complained recently of a change in color of his urine to "a darker shade" which was attributed to dietary intake of soft drinks and red-colored fruit ades. Urine was obtained and revealed the presence of 3+ proteinuria and massive microscopic hematuria with red cell casts easily observed. The urine when obtained was a cloudy orange color, which is common in acute poststreptococcal glomerulonephritis. In this particular instance the physician was immediately directed to the primary diagnosis and was able to manage the hypertension adequately and restore the child to a normotensive level with ensuing complete recovery.

The rapid sorting out of the possible causes of coma in a 6-year-old who is hypertensive illustrates again the necessity for factual knowledge, which will not be further explored. In addition, it illustrates the need to maintain several probable diagnoses in mind, based on the best information available, and to explore these diagnoses while considering secondary possibilities only in screening fashion initially. The clinical scenario in this child could have been altered dramatically if the urine had been clear and the hypertension had been found in the upper extremities, in which case the clinician would have been directed more toward cardiovascular causes, such as coarctation of the aorta. Alternatively, the urine may have been clear, the blood pressure uniform throughout, and the spinal fluid suggestive of encephalitis, in which case the clinician's attention could have been directed in that sphere. The important principle is that the initial steps that the clinician undertook were designed to probe in an urgent way the most probable diagnoses, but allow subsequent steps that might be necessary to establish a diagnosis originally considered at a secondary level.

Case #3

The 15-year-old child in Case #3 represents one end of the spectrum that the clinician must consider whenever he encounters a child who has received head trauma. Trauma to the head is one of the more common accidents that occurs to children, with subsequent effects ranging from insignificant superficial scalp injuries to massive intracranial bleeds. The history most often is of very recent origin, although in some instances many days may supervene between the initial trauma and the clinical manifestations. The clinician must be prepared to sort from the large number of children with cranial injuries who require no diagnostic procedure and no therapy, those who demand immediate diagnostic procedures and/or therapy. To do so requires a recognition of the spectrum and the classic symptoms associated with each of the major intracranial manifestations of trauma, as well as a sound idea of the variations that may be encountered in clinical practice.

In this child the central nervous system symptoms are the most prominent and the most urgent to consider. The child moves rapidly from a confused, dazed state to fairly profound coma with focal manifestations and evidence of severe cerebral insult. There is little time for reflection and careful consideration of all of the alternative possibilities. The clinician must be guided by the clues available and must act with great haste, in that the evolving clinical state appears to be life-threatening. The child has manifestations of shock and of profound cerebral dysfunction, and the clinician must quickly sort through the possibilities, making correct diagnostic and therapeutic choices as he goes. The major handhold for the clinician here is the presence of the dilating pupil occurring in sequence with a rapid alteration in consciousness and in cerebral irritability. The clinician rapidly concludes that the patient has an ipsilateral epidural hematoma, in that these manifestations are classic for this process. Obviously, he must know this and be prepared to identify the eye changes which lead him to this conclusion.

This child did have extradural hematoma, and with rapid diagnosis and neurosurgical consultation the child's shock and blood loss were stabilized and the lesion was evacuated. The critical component that led from an obvious history to identification of the appropriate neurologic changes and a matching of the manifestations with the known mechani-

cal problems that produced them was fracture of the skull rupturing the middle meningeal artery, leading to epidural hematoma.

The evolving coma may have been more slowly paced and may not have had such a classic presentation, in which case the clinician may have had to consider other causes of alteration of consciousness following trauma, such as concussion, subdural hematoma, and subarachnoid hemorrhage. The clinician whose responsibility it is to care for individuals in acute emergent situations must be fully familiar with the classic descriptions of each of these clinical situations and of their common variations. Further, he must adapt himself to the reevaluation, paying particular attention to evolving symptoms and signs and the pace of that evolution.

Case #4

The puzzling presentation in the 10-year-old female in Case #4 can be quickly sorted out if attention is paid to detail. Essentially we have a previously well, well-behaved 10-year-old female whose illness has only been of 1-week's duration and consists of very vague findings, which in themselves are not diagnostic. The additional information that dysuria has been intermittently present and was associated with nocturia tends to implicate the renal system in this child's illness. However, it would be difficult to explain the bizarre behavior and the increasing lethargy, inattentiveness and abdominal pain of vague character on the basis of classic pyelonephritis. It is conceivable that the child has an infectious disorder of the urinary tract which has resulted in gram-negative endotoxic shock to account for the current presentation, but that leaves unexplained her central nervous system findings of more than a week's duration. Faced with this puzzling set of circumstances the clinician must rapidly consider disorders leading to coma that are characterized by this combination of symptoms.

Seeking clues in the physical examination, the physician is hard pressed to identify any characteristic features. Coma and incipient shock are obvious, but her respirations are inconsistent with these grave states. Deep, rapid respirations in the presence of coma suggest metabolic derangement. This could be of primary nature, based on some inherent metabolic abnormality, or could be secondary to renal or pulmonary disease, teleologically resulting in the need for excessive ventilation. This type of pathophysiologic reasoning leads the clinician to consider metabolic and renal causes of coma.

Apart from the dysuria and nocturia of recent onset, the clinician has no reason to suspect prolonged renal disease unless it has been of the silent variety. Nevertheless, one necessary probe to test this hypothesis will be examination of both the urine and blood for alterations that suggest the presence of a chronic renal process, such as pyelonephritis, and for its metabolic derangements that might be attendant upon some degree of renal failure. Alternatively, he will explore metabolic causes, the most prominent of which is diabetes mellitus, which can produce behavioral changes, urinary symptoms, and the vague findings of abdominal pain, lethargy, etc. Thus, in fairly rapid order the clinician has established the priorities of initial hypotheses, and the finding of glycosuria and excess acetone in the urine is not surprising and leads to establishment of the diagnosis of diabetes mellitus and diabetic ketoacidosis as the cause for this child's illness. In addition, she has an acute urinary tract infection, which presumably has precipitated her from the latent to the overt diabetic state.

In this case the clinician has used a pathophysiologic approach to establish the diagnosis. The symptoms are not sufficiently specific to suggest an anatomic localization (save for the possibility of renal disease), nor is any specific etiologic category immediately suggested because of the nonspecificity of the complaints. Thus, the clinician combines vague historical information with physical examination changes that lead him to establish the broad pathophysiologic categories of metabolic and renal disorder as the most probable underlying causes. He might also have considered the possibility of poisoning, either accidental or due to specific drug abuse, which also might have accounted for the acute manifestations. However, he would be hard pressed to explain the week-long illness and the prior normal behavior in a 10-year-old unless there was ancillary evidence that the child had a source of chronic poisoning or a history and personality consistent with drug abuse.

SUMMARY

The comatose child represents a challenge to the diagnostician in both establishment of diagnostic priority and urgency of intercession. Clinical reasoning in this area demands an adequate fund of knowledge to delineate common causes of the production of coma, plus a logical utilization of historical and physical examination data to direct initial diagnostic probes consistent with adequate hypothesis setting. In some instances the hypothesis will be straightforward and single because of the specificity of clues that the patient's history and physical examination provide. In others the comatose state will be accompanied by vague or diffuse symptomatology and findings, and the clinician may find that a pathophysiologic approach is more productive than the anatomic one.

Chapter 10

The Child with Anemia

INTRODUCTION

The child presenting with a lower hemoglobin concentration represents an example of one of the more orderly diagnostic processes that occur in pediatric practice. The system whereby the body produces and maintains adequate oxygen-carrying capacity of the blood is a well ordered and highly regulated one.

Red blood cells are produced in the bone marrow throughout life, in sites of extramedullary hematopoiesis in early life, and occasionally in certain disease states at other ages. Synthesis of red blood cells is dependent upon the availability of protein, certain metalic substrates and other trace elements and on a supply of adequate vitamins to act as cofactors in the various processes. The stimulus for red blood cell production is the level of tissue oxygen, and alterations in production are determined by erythropoietin, a hormone that stimulates red blood cell production. The process of red blood cell production and release from the bone marrow includes a series of steps in which undifferentiated stem cells become mature erythrocytes. This end product cell consists largely of hemoglobin, lasts approximately 120 days in circulation, and has the major function of oxygen transport and release in the tissues.

Circulation of erythrocytes to all tissues is dependent upon an intact circulatory system, and regulation of red cell mass is finally managed by removal of aged erythrocytes in the reticuloendothelial system.

Thus it can be seen that anemia, or reduction in the hemoglobin-carrying capacity, can occur as the result of a faulty production of adequate erythrocytes in adequate numbers, a loss of red blood cells either within the circulating system or by bleeding from it, and, finally, by excessive destruction of red cells reducing the red cell mass below that which the body is capable of producing. Examples of these types of anemia are illustrated by actual case histories below.

CASE HISTORIES

Case #1

A 12-month-old infant is referred to a well-baby clinic because he has not seen a physician and the parents are interested in having him receive immunizations.

A review of the child's past history reveals a normal pregnancy, labor and delivery and an unremarkable first year of life save for frequent respiratory infections within the last month. The child was breast-fed for the first 3 months of life and then received 1 to 2 qt of formula or milk every day thereafter. In addition, his diet was supplemented with rice cereal beginning at 4 months of age, and because he displayed a voracious appetite, fruits were added at 6 months. He has enjoyed that diet to the present with the substitution of table foods most recently, including mashed potatoes, squash and other soft vegetables that could be mashed.

A complete review of systems reveals no abnormalities, and his development has been normal in relation to the usual milestones except that he has not yet walked, which the parents attribute to his being "heavy."

Physical examination of the infant reveals him to be in the 95th percentile for height and weight, and the examiner notes that he is "chubby." The baby has striking pallor, and his skin is described as "thin." He appears irritable to the examiner, with a constant fussiness during the entire period of observation. He has a cloudy mucoid discharge in both nares, but the rest of his physical examination is within normal limits.

Case #2

A 10-month-old child has had a completely uneventful history until 1 month ago. He was the product of a normal pregnancy, labor and delivery, was breast-fed for the first 7 months of life, after which he was given no more than 12 to 14 oz of formula a day fortified with iron, and has been increasingly fed a rich variety of fruits, vegetables and meats by utilizing prepared baby foods.

One month ago he was noticed to become extremely irritable, alternating with periods of lethargy, and his parents observed that he slept more than previous children in their family. Although his stool pattern had been normal prior to 1 month ago, on at least 3 occasions in the past month, mother has noted him to pass sticky, thick, black-brown stools during episodes of extreme irritability which lasted 2 to 3 days each.

Physical examination reveals an extremely pale and very irritable infant who is at the 50th percentile for height and weight. His physical examination is otherwise completely normal.

Case #3

A 6-month-old infant presents with persistent jaundice since the newborn period. His pregnancy was complicated by incompatibility in the ABO system, and the infant developed jaundice and anemia thought to be secondary to the ABO incompatibility,

and two transfusions were performed. The infant's jaundice gradually subsided, and he was discharged at 1 week of age.

His pediatrician thought he was jaundiced at the 2- and 4-month visits but was uncertain. At the 6-month visit he decided to check his clinical suspicions, found the bilirubin level to be 6.5 mg/100 ml, and referred the patient to you.

Family history reveals a Swedish heritage. A number of relatives have gallbladder disease, including some with gallstones who required surgical intervention.

Case #4

A 15-year-old boy is referred to you because of his increasing lethargy and the appearance of purplish spots on his body. His primary physician had diagnosed chronic active hepatitis 1 year ago, and following an initially stormy course in which the hepatitis was documented, a tissue diagnosis of subacute hepatitis with cirrhotic changes was made subsequently.

Since that time he has been maintained with an initial course of steroid therapy, which has been discontinued for the past 9 months, and he has gradually recovered to the point where he is attending school and participating in modest sports and recreational activities. About 2 months ago he began complaining of increasing fatigue and inability to keep up with his classmates. He frequently returned from school in the afternoon and slept until suppertime, which represented an unusual pattern for him.

Within the past several days he has developed a variety of purplish "spots" on his body, and his primary care physician reports that he has both anemia and thrombocytopenia, and he has been referred to you for further diagnosis.

This 15-year-old is muscular and at the 75th percentile for height and weight. His vital signs are normal, and he is afebrile. His physical examination is unremarkable except for an enlarged liver (9 cm) and a large, firm, palpable spleen which extends below the midaxillary line for 3 cm. On his extremities and trunk he has multiple small macular red-blue-purple areas which are nontender and are not affected by pressure. Several of the areas are stated by the patient to be old and have a brownish coloration.

CLINICAL ANALYSIS

With the knowledge that most anemias can be accounted for by deficient production or excessive destruction or loss, the clinician approaching a child in whom anemia is suspected can follow a fairly orderly thought sequence. The history should be carefully ascertained for the duration of symptoms, for dietary habits which might suggest undernutrition or specific nutrient deficiencies, for rate of growth, and for evidence of blood loss or excessive destruction of red blood cells with production of bilirubin leading to jaundice. In addition, the family history should be carefully surveyed for other examples suggestive of the same disease process in the child. Finally, the history should be sifted for any evidence of other disease manifestations which might have anemia as one component.

The physical examination is directed towards establishment of low hemoglobin, with the color of skin and mucous membranes carefully noted, and for the presence of jaundice, which may be indicative of excessive red cell destruction. In addition, evidence of other disease should be sought, and the spleen palpated for carefully.

Armed with historical and physical examination data, the clinician then systematically searches for the combination of data that suggests deficient production or excessive destruction of red blood cells. Deficient production would be suggested by an inadequate dietary intake leading to protein or a specific nutrient deficiency, such as lack of iron in the diet. When such a history is coupled with the observation of pallor, weakness and other signs of inadequate oxygenation in the infant or child, suspicion of anemia is aroused, and specific probes can then be made. Excessive destruction or loss is suggested by evidence of hemorrhage or more subtle blood loss, or by the external manifestations of jaundice, or by the presence of characteristics of a variety of disease states which may be associated with excessive red cell destruction (such as splenomegaly).

The first task confronting the clinician is to establish the degree and type of anemia.

For this determination the clinician utilizes the so-called hematologic indices, which include hemoglobin, hematocrit and total red blood cell count, and the derived mean corpuscular hemoglobin, mean corpuscular volume, and mean corpuscular hemoglobin concentration. Also essential in this initial determination is examination of the peripheral blood smear for both the nature and character of normal erythrocytes and for the presence of aberrant forms.

In this case the clinician can fairly easily establish the presence or absence of anemia. In itself, this is a relatively simple diagnostic task and does not require extensive diagnostic prowess. In fact, because of the presence of minor degrees of anemia throughout childhood, it has been suggested that part of well-child care consist of periodic assessment of hemoglobin and hematocrit as a screening device to pick up those individuals who have asymptomatic or mildly symptomatic anemia. A more challenging diagnostic process begins following the establishment of anemia as the homeostatic state of the individual. In this endeavor the clinician is seeking to determine the specific cause of the anemia, rather than seeking simply to describe its presence.

In Case #1 the physical examination strongly suggests to the clinician that the child is anemic. Historically, the setting is one in which dietary intake appears to be inadequate for iron. The consumption of large amounts of milk and carbohydrates in the diet without an adequate source of dietary iron, or with no supplementation of medicinal iron, results in inadequate hemoglobin production and resultant iron deficiency anemia in the latter half of the first year of life or in the second year of life. In this case the clinician can rapidly establish the presence of iron deficiency anemia, utilizing the simple screening test approach. This child had a hemoglobin of 10.0 gm, an hematocrit of 31%, and a microcytic hypochromic red blood cell pattern on smear.

Although the cause seemed self-evident in the dietary history, the clinician searched for any possible blood loss in this infant both historically and by examination of several stools for the presence of blood.

Thus, in straightforward fashion an iron deficiency anemia was established as the primary diagnosis, with nutritional inadequacy of iron intake as the proximate cause. Replacement of dietary iron rapidly resolved the issue in the clinician's mind, and the child was returned to normal hemoglobin levels over the next several months. Counseling of the parents in terms of iron intake and dietary suggestions resulted in a more adequate diet in relation to iron, and the problem was resolved satisfactorily.

This straightforward scenario occurs repeatedly in pediatric practice and requires little more than simple screening tests and the institution of appropriate intervention. On occasion, however, the clinician will be mistaken in attributing the apparent iron deficiency anemia to inadequate dietary intake. A small percentage of these children have chronic blood loss via a gastrointestinal (GI) lesion, which may not be detected by random examination of the stool for occult blood. One notable example in our experience occurred in a child who was treated repeatedly for iron deficiency anemia until she announced rather dramatically that she had a Meckel's diverticulum by the massive outpouring of blood into the GI tract. Her blood loss prior to this had been minimal and intermittent and had escaped detection by random stool analysis for occult blood.

Another infant similarly was treated for apparent iron deficiency anemia on the basis of inadequate intake until events dictated that true milk allergy was present, in that a fairly massive GI bleed was followed by investigation of milk sensitivity, and it was discovered that the infant's blood loss and anemia could be corrected by withholding cow's milk from the diet. No amount of iron supplementation in either of the latter cases made any difference, and although the clinical picture and the initial laboratory data suggested iron deficiency anemia, the true cause was blood loss. This latter must always be borne in mind, although only a very few of the children with characteristic iron deficiency anemia histories will, in fact, have chronic blood loss.

Case #2 illustrates a straightforward example of blood loss anemia which mimicked iron deficiency anemia in many respects. The initial hemoglobin, hematocrit and blood smear were all suggestive of iron deficiency anemia, but the history was incompatible with excessive milk intake, and the diet appeared to be adequate in iron-containing fluids and food.

The episodes of irritability and change in the character of stools strongly suggested the presence of a bleeding GI lesion, although examination for occult blood at the time the child was seen was negative. This child had a duplication of the GI tract in which the adjacent aberrant intestine contained gastric mucosa which had ulcerated and bled intermittently, resulting in the anemia.

The clue here was obviously the presence of black, tarry stools, although, as has been pointed out above, the bleeding may be of minor character without such dramatic change in the stool pattern. In these cases the clinician must establish anemia as the primary diagnosis and consider both inadequate production and blood loss concomitantly.

The degree to which a diligent search is made for the origin of blood loss in the GI tract is partially dependent upon clinical clues, which may or may not be present, and on the discrepancy between the laboratory findings and historical information. We have seen a number of children who have been diagnosed as iron deficiency anemia on an excessive milk intake basis whose histories were incompatible with excessive milk intake. Thus, whenever the clinician encounters a discrepancy between expected history and the actual data in the presence of iron deficiency anemia, chronic GI blood loss must be considered.

Case #3 is more difficult of analysis. In this child the initial screening revealed hemoglobin and hematocrit which were reduced, but the blood smear and indices were indicative of hemolysis. The presence of questionable jaundice was verified with a serum bilirubin level just slightly above 6 mg/100 ml, the level at which skin jaundice can be detected.

The blood smear revealed microcytic hyperchromic cells with a mean corpuscular volume of 75 and a mean corpuscular hemoglobin concentration of 37. Fewer than

10% of the cells on the initial smear were thought to be spherocytes. The reticulocyte count in this instance was elevated (5%), which is a marked contradistinction to most instances of iron deficiency anemia. In this child the smear was critical in that the presence of hyperchromic cells and spherocytes dictated further laboratory analyses to establish whether or not the spherocytic form of congenital hemolytic anemia or hereditary spherocytosis was present. Osmotic fragility tests were performed on the infant's red blood cells and were found to be increased after incubation at 37° for 24 hours. This increased osmotic fragility was corrected with the addition of glucose and adenosine triphosphate, further establishing the defect. The family history of gallbladder disease was suggestive but not necessarily diagnostic. In fact, analysis of the family subsequently determined that a number of mild instances of spherocytosis were present.

In Case #4, the antecedent disease, chronic active hepatitis, had resulted in cirrhotic changes in the liver and to secondary hypersplenism. This child's spleen systematically removed red blood cells and platelets from the circulation to the point that he had anemia and thrombocytopenia of sufficient degree to produce the symptoms and signs recorded. Anemia in this case was a secondary manifestation attributable to excessive removal of normal erythrocytes by a disturbed splenic function secondary to the preexistent hepatic disease.

GENERALIZATIONS

In the diagnosis of anemia in infancy and childhood it is critical to consider the following steps: (1) identification of the anemia, (2) characterization of the anemia and (3) detailed characterization of the type of anemia.

Identification of the Anemia

Whether the identification is because of historical or physical examination data suggestive of its presence, or because of screening of population groups in which anemia has a reasonable frequency, the first step in the diagnostic process is to establish its presence. Usually this is accomplished by the use of the hemoglobin, hematocrit and a simple stained blood smear. The hemoglobin and hematocrit establish the degree of anemia, and the smear may be a clue as to its underlying character. At this point in the diagnostic process the clinician can simply state that anemia is present, and the beginning suspicion of its general origin may be possible. Thus we can say an individual has mild, moderate or severe anemia depending on the degree of variation of hemoglobin from the expected norm for the age, and we may be able to make an initial estimate of whether it is decreased production or excessive destruction that underlies the anemia.

Characterization of the Anemia

Characterization of the anemia, a critical step, is often omitted, especially in iron deficiency anemia, when the identification step appears to indicate clearly iron deficiency anemia. In efficient diagnosis this may be a cost-saving step for most children with straightforward nutritional anemia. It has the inherent danger of missing a few children whose origin of anemia is other than nutritional deficiency. A more complete analysis would include calculation of the indices to verify what is seen on smear, and the addition of a reticulocyte count to add further strength to the assumption that this is a nondestructive anemic process. If either of these determinations are aberrant, i.e., are not consistent with a microcytic hyperchromic anemia without reticulocyte response, the clinician should continue the characterization.

Detailed Characterization of the Type of Anemia

The use of serum iron and iron-binding capacity determinations and examination of the stools for blood are the simplest steps to be taken at this level. In addition, serum protein determination, particularly for those elements associated with red cells, and examination of the bone marrow may be necessary. These steps are carried out if hypochromic anemia is established. The serum ferritin level and free erythrocyte protoporphyrin often are useful in differentiating iron deficiency anemia from other causes of hyperchromic anemic states.

If the smear is hyperchromic (or normochromic), the reticulocyte count becomes an essential determinant. A high reticulocyte count usually indicates hemolytic disease or acute blood loss. In the absence of acute blood loss, the smear should be carefully examined for the presence of abnormal cells, and a Coombs' test should be performed to rule out the possibility of an autoimmune process. Selective use of osmotic fragility testing and the use of hemoglobin electrophoresis may be essential to sort out specific instances of the types of hemolytic anemia. The most sophisticated level of determination is to examine the red cells for their enzyme composition to detect those rare disorders in which enzymatic deficiency results in excessive hemolysis. If the reticulocyte count is low, one must look to the bone marrow with the idea that diminished production or release may be responsible for the normochromic anemia.

Thus, in orderly fashion the clinician can begin with a clinical suspicion and end with a very specific etiologic diagnosis based on a sequential analysis. The use of simple, readily available tests initially, and more complicated maneuvers subsequently, in a series of steps, ultimately leads to delineation of the specific defect.

Chapter 11

The Child with Headache

INTRODUCTION

Headache is one of the most difficult symptom complexes for the pediatrician to evaluate. In early infancy and childhood, headache is distinctly uncommon and may herald very serious disease. As the child progresses through school and the adolescent years, headache becomes more common a complaint, but the overall incidence of serious disease diminishes. Folklore, home remedies and the commonness of headache as a symptom all contribute to delay or neglect in bringing the symptom to the attention of the physician. Even with serious underlying disease in which headache is the primary or sole manifestation, seldom, if ever, is the physician confronted by the patient early in the course. The diagnostic reasoning in headache poses the classical dilemma to the clinician, that of discerning the few individuals who have a serious and even correctable cause from among the very many who display the symptom in which the etiology is transient, trivial or undetectable.

Further complicating the analysis of headache is the subjective nature of pain. No one has been able to measure adequately the degree of discomfort which we refer to as pain. Individual reactivity to such a symptom, and individual tolerance, are reflected in the individual who has a very serious disorder which should produce severe pain but in which the complaint is minimal. Similarly, in an individual with an undetectable, trivial or transient cause of headache, the complaint may far exceed the seriousness of the etiology. This confounding variable often makes it difficult for the physician to evaluate the "quantity" of pain in relation to the need for extensive diagnostic procedures and therapy.

Increasing the diagnostic difficulty is the inability of many young children to describe accurately such characteristics of headache as onset, localization and the precise nature of the pain. One young, preschool child in whom headache was a major complaint simply placed his hands over his entire scalp and said, "It hurts!" in response to any question attempting to define the symptom further. In contrast, many adolescents with recurrent headaches will give detailed descriptions of each of the characteristics which do not follow any anatomic or physiologic pattern that is discernible. Often the precision with which the headache is described suggests to the clinician a serious underlying organic etiology, when in fact the psychologic difficulty producing the headache is also responsible for the almost obsessive quality of the description of each of its characteristics.

In this chapter we will consider the approach to the child with a headache and attempt to delineate those maneuvers which the clinician can employ to identify correctable and serious organic problems from correctable and serious psychologic ones. Each end of the spectrum is important, and one must guard against the attitude that treats as significant only those headaches that have a serious organic mechanism.

THE ETIOLOGY OF HEADACHE IN CHILDREN

In this discussion we will attempt to differentiate the single acute episode of headache from those which have a recurrent pattern. This is a convenient clinical distinction inasmuch as etiology may vary considerably between the two groups. It is important, however, to remember that all recurrent headaches begin as a single acute episode. It is also important to remember that the causes of most headaches are unclear. In some instances, changes in vascular flow to the brain or to structures in the scalp appear to be responsible for the sensation of headache. In fact, we know very little about the connection between the perception of pain in the head and the underlying mechanisms. In most instances, associations are made on the basis of logic; i.e., an expanding pulsatile tumor appears to logically result in pain because of its compression and stretching of intracranial structures. On the other hand, a similar degree of pain may be produced without any evidence of compression or stretching, and therefore the mechanism is probably not that simple.

As mentioned previously, headache in the young child is usually associated with a specific, and often serious, underlying cause. That is, headaches which are unassociated with acute illnesses are often associated with serious underlying disease. It is true that most transient, acute headaches in infants and children are probably the results of acute infections about the head and neck, or acute infections which are associated with serious systemic disturbances, such as fever or "generalized" toxicity. Children old enough to vocalize complaints will often indicate that their head hurts at the same time that they have tonsillopharyngitis, nasorhinitis or otitis media. In these children the headache seems trivial in relation to the more localized pain associated with their infection. Many febrile children, from whatever cause, will complain about diffuse, moderate headache during the periods that they are febrile. This is often accompanied by a generalized feeling of "achiness," and the headache may be described as constant and pounding in nature. In contrast, the slightly older child with well-developed sinuses may complain of head pain localized to the area of sinusitis. For example, the school age child or teenager with acute frontal sinusitis will often experience excruciating headache localized over the frontal area. They often will place their hand or finger over a small area on the forehead to indicate the location of maximum intensity to their pain. Similarly, maxillary sinusitis will often produce excruciating pain over the face, often extending into the orbit. Individuals with mastoiditis will complain of headache localized posterior to the ear and spreading over the scalp on either side. Children who have dental disease of the upper teeth may experience excruciating pain, often described as "piercing," radiating in the facial and lower scalp areas.

In contrast to most folklore, excessive reading, reading in a poor light, refractive disorders, and other ocular abnormalities rarely are responsible for the headaches observed in children who also display these phenomena. Although the temporal association of a great deal of reading and headache seems logical to the layman as evidence of causation, it is often forgotten that other factors, such as the tension of the task for which the reading is being done, fatigue, or concomitant respiratory illness, may actually be responsible. In younger children, acute, severe headache, often localized to one area of the cranial vault, may be indicative of intracranial mass lesions. In contrast to the more diffuse headaches associated with acute inflammatory disease, this type of headache tends to be persistent and progressive in character. Often, vomiting accompanies the headache, and associated symptomatology may also be observed. Ataxia, excessive irritability, aimless activity, and frequent change of posture have been reported in such children. Frequently, sudden change in posture will exacerbate the headache and often will produce unbearable pain. When quizzed, children with this type of headache often will localize it to one portion of the scalp consistently. Although it is said that the location of headache may be diagnostic of the location of the underlying tumor, there are enough instances in which this does not occur that the clinician should not rely upon it.

In some children with obstructive lesions to the flow of spinal fluid, the onset of acute hydrocephalus may be heralded by acute headache. In many such children, other signs of the underlying cause of the obstruction will be more evident than the symptom of headache. On the other hand, some children have progressive closure of spinal fluid flow, and headache may be the sole or primary manifestation in the early stages of the process. In our section of the country, the Southwest desert, meningitis due to coccidioidomycosis, a fungus found in our region, can produce acute hydrocephalus. Children commonly present with headache, vomiting, and ataxia in any combination. On the other hand, children with tuberculous meningitis in which hydrocephalus is a prominent feature will often have many manifestations prior to the onset of headache.

An infrequent occurrence in pediatric practice, but one that is important to remember, is the increase in intracranial pressure unassociated with obstruction of spinal fluid flow or any mass lesion within the cranial vault. This is so-called benign intracranial hypertension or pseudotumor cerebri. In pediatrics it most commonly is associated with otitis media and has been termed otitic hydrocephalus. In addition, drugs, including the tetracyclines, the steroid compounds, and excessive vitamin A intake, may produce the syndrome. In adolescent and older children it may be part of the symptom complex of acute lupus erythematosus. Further, it has been associated with excessive obesity and with irregularities in the menstrual cycle, often as part of the complex of premenstrual syndromes.

Rarely, other types of cerebral masses, apart from benign and malignant tumors, may produce headache. Of these, brain abscess and subdural collections are the most common. In these disorders, although headache may be a prominent feature, there usually are many other signs and symptoms accompanying the underlying disorder. On rare occasions, headache may be the only and primary symptom early in the course of abscess or subdural collection.

Trauma in childhood is a common experience. Acute headache following a blow to the head is self-explanatory. However, many children who experience the concussion syndrome as a result of acute trauma will develop headache at some point thereafter. It is not uncommon for a child who has experienced a concussion to complain of acute headache for some days or even weeks after the injury. This type of headache is usually localized to the site of injury and is very persistent. Other children will manifest a recurrent pattern of headache, which will be discussed later. One must be prepared to accept the secondary gain that such symptoms may have for the child whose initial injury achieved a great deal of attention and sympathy. If the child's family and psychologic circumstances are such that sustenance of symptomatology will appear to benefit the value with which he or she is held, headache may become a very valuable asset, and the symptom may unconsciously be exaggerated.

In older children the so-called tension headache may occur for the first time and is believed to be related to sustained contraction of the paraspinal muscles. Although these headaches tend to be recurrent in nature, the first episode is often brought to the clinician's attention because of the details provided by the sufferer. Often this is an adolescent girl who is slightly obese with a history of nervousness or behavioral disorder in the past. The headache is described as band-like and constant, but attempts to define it further are often impossible. The child may place a hand over the neck in expressing a portion of the symptomatology and, according to Dr. Peggy Ferry, our Child Neurologist, almost invariably will pinch the bridge of the nose, pressing the hand deep into the sockets in describing the pain. Dr. Ferry feels that this kind of sign is almost never seen in other types of headache.

There are other causes of acute headache in children which are so infrequent as not to merit discussion here. Almost all children with the acute onset of headache will fit into one of the patterns above. In a few of these instances the headache will become progressive or recurrent, and these phenomena merit separate discussion.

PROGRESSIVE OR RECURRENT HEADACHES

In the child who has had cerebral trauma, headache may result from a variety of causes. First, the headache may occur at the site of injury after an interval and be persistent. The cause for this type of headache has never been delineated, but it is one of the more difficult syndromes to deal with. It may be related to subtle injury to the sensory nerves supplying the area that was traumatized. The persistent headache is occasionally debilitating but is most often just inconvenient to the patient. Some children will complain of inability to concentrate and often require excessive analgesic efforts in an attempt to relieve the pain. In this syndrome the pain tends to occur at the site of injury, and its duration is extremely variable; in some children, only a few days of discomfort is experienced, and in others many months may pass before the symptom disappears.

In the child who sustained original trauma, an undiagnosed subdural hematoma may result. As the hematoma undergoes its physiologic repair, osmotic pressures may be generated which increase its size, and the expansion of the lesion may result in headache. These children most commonly have other manifestations, such as focal neurologic disturbances or convulsions, or even fever, as a more prominent symptom than headache. In some, headache will be the primary manifestation or will be part of a complex involving these other phenomena. The headache is usually localized to the site of the subdural hematoma or to its referral pattern onto the scalp.

Children who have other types of mass intracranial lesions tend to have progressive headache that increases in severity prior to discovery and treatment of the lesion. Characteristically the headache will be localized to one area of the scalp and will increase in intensity and often reach a level in which total disability is experienced. In some children, diffuse generalized head pain with pre-

dominance in the frontal or occipital area will be characteristic. As indicated previously, associated symptoms of vomiting, irritability, aimless movements, and frequent changes in posture may all accompany this kind of headache. Depending on the localization of the tumor, specific neurologic symptoms may develop. For example, in tumors of the cerebellum and posterior fossa, ataxia may be a prominent feature.

Other types of recurrent headaches include three major syndromes: pediatric migraine, tension syndrome, and occipital neuralgia. In addition, particularly in adolescence, headache may reflect serious underlying psychologic disorder. Depression, hysterical conversion reactions, serious malingering, and other severe personality disorders may express themselves initially as headaches. In any individual child a pattern to the occurrence and description of the headache may be developed which is really symptomatic of the more serious behavioral disorganization that produced it.

Pediatric migraine differs somewhat from the adult pattern. In children, migraine tends to be bilateral, in contrast to the unilateral form in adults. It often is frontal in localization, and it is described by the child as pulsating in character. Frequently, severe abdominal discomfort appears more prominent than headache in children. This is uncommon in adults. The child often appears ill, and this component is often of such degree that the child seeks solitude and wants to be left alone until the symptoms pass. Parents often describe the child as holding the abdomen and lying quietly in a darkened room, avoiding all contact with others insofar as possible. Also characteristic is the onset of sleep, once the attack subsides. Parents frequently will describe this as unusual for the child. Initial episodes are often attributed to some acute gastrointestinal upset. It is only with the recurrence of the symptomatology that the parents bring the child to a physician's attention. Less commonly than adults, children may experience an aura, but the classical scotomata and paresthesias are distinctly less common in childhood than they are in the adult pattern. As the symptoms persist, a more classic adult pattern may be observed, and any of the various adult migraine patterns may develop. It is beyond the scope of this text to discuss migraine in more detail, and the reader is referred to neurologic and pediatric sources.

So-called tension headaches are the most common cause of recurrent headaches in childhood. In some children they appear to be a somatization of chronic anxiety, and in others they are a forerunner and herald of serious underlying personality disorders. They tend to recur at irregular intervals, and diligent historical search often elicits a specific stressful situation as provoking for the symptomatology. In contrast with children with migraine, children with recurring tension headaches seldom have their activity interfered with. Of course, if the tension of the moment is related to a particular school or family situation, the headache may serve to assist the child in avoiding that particular stress. However, simultaneously, recreational or other activities will not be interfered with. Tension headache may also occur as a result of prolonged activity leading to fatigue contraction of the cervical paraspinal muscles. A diligent student who spends hours bent over a typewriter, preparing a final theme, may find occipital headache one unexpected result. In such individuals the activity itself may be the predisposing cause, or a combination of tension plus the prolonged activity.

Occipital neuralgia is a specific syndrome delineated in the 1950's whose incidence is difficult to establish. It is believed to be related to instability of the joint space between the first and second cervical vertebrae, resulting in subluxation of the joint and compression of the spinal nerves exiting. These children will often tilt the head away from the side of the pain and will complain of severe occipital pain, often localized to the muscles on that side of the neck. Some neurologists and orthopedists consider other aberrations of the cervical spine with compression of exiting spinal nerve roots as a cause of persistent headache in some children. These are often difficult to prove, and convincing evidence for the actual mechanism is often not possible.

The exploration of the mechanisms of pain by modern specialists has led to the belief that there are some individuals with musculofascial areas of increased irritability, so-called "trigger points." Some of these trigger points are located in and about the posterior neck and, when they are compressed, will produce a classic pattern of pain for that patient. Often the pain is of headache quality and characteristics. It frequently is occipital, radiates over the posterior scalp, and is associated with localized tenderness and even paresthesias. Although better delineated in adults, many physicians believe that older children and adolescents may also experience this type of pain. Frequently the symptoms can be reproduced by point pressure or insertion of a needle into the trigger-point area. Relief is often sustained by injection of local anesthetics or steroid compounds into the area. The current belief is that these are areas of localized inflammation in the muscle for reasons that are not clear.

In addition to these classic syndromes of recurrent headache in children, a large number of syndromes and patterns are observed in individuals which cannot be attributed to any distinct cause. In many such children, allergic manifestations in other organ systems may have been present for some time. Some allergists and pediatricians believe that the headaches are related to allergy in some fashion, and that the target organ is the cerebral vasculature rather than the nose, skin or lung. This association is extremely difficult to prove and almost as difficult to manage.

Some recurrent headaches are related to serious underlying personality disorders. It is beyond the scope of this chapter, however, to explore the relationship of headache to such mental states as depression, hysteria and malingering. Of pertinence to us is recognition that headache may be the sole manifestation of such states, and in our approach to be described, adequate psychologic assessment is necessary.

Some recurrent headaches in older children and adolescents may occur as a result of environmental influences, such as the inhalation or ingestion of noxious substances. Individuals exposed to sublethal doses of carbon monoxide repetitively, for example, may experience recurrent headaches until the source is identified and eliminated. Similarly, children who abuse drugs may experience headache after such episodes, related pharmacologically to the agents they utilized or to the concomitant personality characteristics which led them to drug abuse in the first place. For example, a child with depressive tendencies who abuses amphetamine type drugs may experience severe headaches in periods of nondrug use. The headache may be related to the pharmacologic recovery from amphetamines or may be related to underlying depression for which the amphetamine abuse was sought. These types of occurrence of headache are sufficiently varied and individualized that their only value in our discussion here is to indicate that they do occur and will assist us in determining the kind of historical and physical examination approach we will utilize.

THE DIAGNOSTIC APPROACH TO THE CHILD WITH HEADACHE

Armed with the knowledge of age relatedness of the various headache syndromes, the clinician will begin his analysis with a precise definition of the headache. In the older child, and with certain of the syndromes above, a very clear-cut pattern of headache will emerge. Such factors as the mode of onset, the duration of the headache, the progressive or nonprogressive quality of the pain, the duration of the individual headache symptom, the association with environmental and other factors, the presence or absence of associated symptoms and signs, and the impact that the headache has on other activities will all assist the clinician in delineating a precise pattern. Unfortunately, in young infants and children such definition may be impossible. The subjective nature of the symptoms and the child's inability to articulate adequately some of the features it would be desirable to delineate result in a "fuzzy" description at best.

Nevertheless, the clinician should make every attempt in his initial assessment to carefully detail every characteristic possible of the headache. As can be seen from consideration of the descriptions of the various headache symptoms, historical delineation in itself may strongly suggest the correct hypothesis to the diagnostician. In such instances the physical examination and laboratory inquiry can be directed appropriately and swiftly to confirm the diagnostic impression formed on the basis of historical facts.

In instances in which the history is not revealing of the underlying nature of the cause of headaches, the physical examination may yield valuable information. Evidence for focal, dental or respiratory disease and "hard" neurologic signs, particularly involvement of the cranial nerves or disturbances in motor or equilibrium function, may provide clues to the origin of the headache. All children with headache deserve a very careful physical examination with particular attention to the nervous system. In addition, blood pressure should be obtained in such fashion as to assess for hypertension accurately. Hypertensive headaches are uncommon in children but can be simply detected by means of accurate assessment of blood pressure.

A general assessment of the child's development, both physically and cognitively, should be made, particularly in instances of prolonged or recurrent headaches. Chronic infections and some malignancies, such as craniopharyngioma, may be suggested by retardation in physical growth or delayed development. Visual acuity should be assessed, particularly if mass lesions of the anterior fossa are suspected.

Adequate examination of the fontanels and of the optic discs is essential in every child with headache. Obviously, abnormalities here can provide clues to increased intracranial pressure. In children with headache the examination is not complete unless the optic discs have been adequately visualized, and this may require dilatation of the pupils.

If the physician has completed the history and physical examination and does not have specific hypotheses in mind, nonspecific assessment of intracranial mechanics is in order. Since subtle increased intracranial pressure may be present in some syndromes, it would be unwise to proceed to a lumbar puncture at this stage for fear of herniation. Rather, the clinician should assess the child by means of skull X-ray or computerized axial tomographic scan. The diagnostic approach is in response to the hypothesis that increased intracranial pressure may be present and may be detected by either of these procedures.

Further diagnostic analysis is obviously dependent on the hypotheses formed at this stage. If one has no reason to suspect serious intracranial disorders, it is unwise to proceed with elaborate, expensive and potentially damaging investigations. For example, if the tension headache syndrome has been delineated by history and physical examination, further diagnostic procedures are unwarranted at that stage. Rather, a more elaborate history should be obtained, perhaps with the help of other professionals, such as clinical psychologists or psychiatrists, rather than pursuit of unlikely and improbable organic causes.

In this regard, careful investigation of the child's family and school or other environments is essential. In many instances it is necessary to separate the parents and the child and take separate histories in order to elicit information that might not be achievable with both parties present.

After initial hypothesis setting and testing, the diagnostic pathway may follow many different courses, depending on the individual characteristics of headache analysis for each child. It is beyond the scope of this chapter to detail the application of such techniques as arteriography, pneumoencephalography and other such studies. In fact, it would be impossible to do so, since individual patterns are sufficiently varied that the precise diagnostic techniques utilized will be largely dependent on the current status of the child and the sequential findings on laboratory tests. The clinician must keep in mind that he is sorting out serious, correctable or approachable lesions in both the organic and psychologic spheres from among the many headache syndromes that are transient, that do not require elaborate diagnostic procedures, and that are responsive to relatively simple measures.

As has been emphasized previously, the most critical element is an adequate history and physical examination delineating the pattern in an individual child. Most hypotheses can be established early in the course of diagnostic analysis, and although a few individual circumstances will defy any diagnostic approach, many, if not most, will yield to this type of sequential reasoning. The greatest mistake that a diagnostician can make is to take the symptom of headache for granted and not delineate its character further and then to proceed through the list of differential diagnosis possibilities, ignoring the probability that could be established with more accurate definition. In such instances the clinician may employ unnecessary and even dangerous diagnostic techniques to a problem that does not merit such exploration. At the very least, the patient may be inconvenienced, both financially and in terms of comfort, and at the very worst, considerable damage can be done, both physically and psychologically, by excessive focus on highly improbable causes for the symptom.

Chapter 12

Recurrent Infections in Infants and Children

INTRODUCTION

In contrast to acute problems considered in other chapters, the child with recurrent infections presents a slowly evolving situation which requires initial assessment and periodic reassessment. The clinical reasoning employed in this situation is a combination of evaluation of each acute episode plus a more comprehensive analysis of the child's entire clinical history. Consideration of the child with recurrent infections allows us to examine diagnostic reasoning in a setting in which multiple factors must be taken into account, including frequency, sequence, character and cause of individual episodes. In addition, the clinician must utilize genetic and family information, measurements of growth and development of the child, and assessment of the child's response to the individual infections. Thus this is a complex set of analyses, and much less straightforward than some of the problems previously considered.

CASE HISTORIES

The difficulties to be encountered can be summarized and exemplified by two complete case histories.

Case #1

An 11-month-old male child was born to a family in which four previous pregnancies had yielded three normal females and one normal male. His pregnancy, labor and delivery were uncomplicated, as was his newborn period and the first 3 months of infancy. He fed well, appeared to be developing normally, and had received his first childhood immunizations at 2 months of age without difficulty. In his fourth month of life he began to develop a series of acute infections that can best be characterized by the following sequence:

Age	Acute Episode
3½ months	Upper respiratory tract infection (URI), febrile
4 months	Diarrhea
4¾ months	URI
5 months	URI with fever and convulsion
5½ months	Diarrhea
6½ months	URI with otitis media
7 months	URI with otitis media
7½ months	URI
7¾ months	URI
8¾ months	Diarrhea
9 months	Pneumonia
10½ months	URI
11 months	Pneumonia

This, then, was the history presented to the physician at the time the child was first seen by the consultant at 11 months of age. The questions asked of the consultant were, Is this child immunodeficient? If the child is immunodeficient, is this a B-cell deficiency?

Case #2

A 12-month-old male had his illnesses begin at 4½ months of age. Prior to that time he was perfectly normal, and he was the first-born child to 18-year-old parents. His pregnancy, labor and delivery were uncomplicated, and the first 4½ months of life were normal. Mother elected to breast-feed the infant and had just begun to supplement him with rice cereal and fruits when he developed his first episode. His pattern can be characterized as follows:

Age	Acute Episode
4½ months	Pneumonia
5 months	URI, fever, conjunctivitis
6 months	Pneumonia
6½ months	Diarrhea, fever, convulsion
7 months	Conjunctivitis
7½ months	Pneumonia
8 months	URI with otitis media
8½ months	URI with otitis media
8¾ months	Pneumonia
9 months	URI with otitis media (the physician thought he had chronic changes in both tympanic membranes)
9½ months	Pneumonia
10 months	Impetigo, conjunctivitis, URI and otitis
10½ months	Diarrhea
11 months	Pneumonia
12 months	Pneumonia, conjunctivitis, otitis media

It was at this last episode that the consultant was asked to see the child, with the same questions posed as in Case #1.

ANALYSES

In both cases presented, it is apparent that marked similarities are present. At least superficially, these two children look alike, and should the data end with only that described, it would be very difficult to distinguish the two case histories. At this point the clinician must probe, adding additional historical information and physical examination data in a systematic fashion. In order to do so, he must clearly understand the genesis of recurrent infections in infants and children and those factors that can assist him in sorting out the truly immunodeficient child from all others.

Let us look at Case #1 in a great deal more detail. The descriptives used by the primary care physician do not tell us a great deal about the character of each infectious epi-

sode. As has been pointed out elsewhere, precise and clearly described data are essential to the problem-solving process. If one accepts the diagnoses at face value, it becomes extremely difficult to determine whether significant underlying disease exists. However, as we shall see, careful delineation of such terms as "upper respiratory tract infection" and "diarrhea" will aid immeasurably in giving these manifestations appropriate weight in our ultimate analysis. When quizzed, the parents volunteered the information that most of the URIs consisted of an afebrile, clear, watery discharge that lasted for 2 or 3 days and was accompanied by anorexia and irritability of mild degree. On only a few occasions was fever actually present, the most notable of which was the episode at 5 months of age, which was accompanied by a febrile convulsion. On the other hand, diarrhea, as described by these parents, consisted of 5 to 6 watery stools on 1 or 2 days, unassociated with blood, mucus, or much discomfort on the part of the infant. The parents could lend no further information concerning the diagnosis of otitis media and pneumonia, since to them these episodes resembled URIs previously described. Later on, the primary care physician was contacted, and he volunteered the information that the otitis media consisted largely of redness of the tympanic membrane and some distortion of the landmarks but no frank bulging, and at no time did he feel there was pus behind the eardrums. Pneumonia consisted of his hearing rales bilaterally in this infant at a time when he was febrile with an URI. His notes reveal there was little cough at the time, and only mild respiratory distress with a transient tachypnea was noted for 2 to 3 days in each episode.

What now emerges from this further data collection is that the episodes were unlikely to be bacterial in origin and in several instances might have represented noninfectious etiology. At least several of the upper respiratory tract episodes were without fever and lasted for brief periods of time. The primary care physician further volunteered that although he had cultured the child's respiratory and intestinal secretions at several points during the course, he had abandoned doing so, since none of the cultures isolated a significant pathogen. However, he did treat most of the episodes with either ampicillin or erythromycin and, in his own mind, associated clearing with the administration of antibiotics.

In Case #2, in contrast, the further history revealed quite a different pattern. In each instance of pneumonia described the child was noted to have high fever, prominent cough, and moderate to marked respiratory distress. The URIs were always accompanied by fever and, on the last several instances, with a marked bilateral otitis media with bulging eardrums. At 9 months of age, the clinician was convinced, chronic changes had already occurred, in that both eardrums appeared to be scarred and thickened. Each episode was treated with antibiotics, blindly initially, but on four occasions pneumococcus had been grown from the blood during the febrile episode, and in all instances of conjunctivitis the pneumococcus was grown from ocular specimens. In the current episode, *Hemophilus influenzae* Type B was isolated from the blood, and pneumococcus was isolated from the ocular pus. The two episodes of diarrhea were bloody, with abundant mucoid discharge and abundant polymorphonuclear leukocytes seen on smear of a rectal swab. In one instance no bacterial pathogen was identified, and in the other, *Shigella sonnei* was isolated.

Already the clinician is beginning to draw a distinction between the two case histories. In the first child it is apparent that the frequent and repetitive infections appear to be nonbacterial in origin and may even be noninfectious, at least in some instances. In contrast, the second child had clearly diagnosed bacterial infections with pyogenic bacteria and of a moderate to severe character.

The diagnostician armed with these additional data begins to develop a quite different mental set in regards to underlying etiology. Before we proceed with the analyses, it would be useful to digress for a moment and consider the causes of chronic recurrent infections in infancy.

RECURRING INFECTIONS IN INFANCY

For most normal infants the occurrence of infectious diseases is a relatively minor part of life. Family studies have shown that children under 6 may have as many as 6 to 12 infectious episodes a year, almost always of minor character and typically consisting of an URI secondary to one of the respiratory or enteric viruses. These normal children have no underlying pathophysiologic disorder, and simply are expressing their additional contact with a multitude of infectious agents by a brisk inflammatory response. This type of infection follows the usual normal distribution curve, in that some infants will breeze through infancy with no or virtually no episodes, whereas others will appear to be ill almost constantly with a new infectious agent. Characteristically, these infections are mild and self-limited, are almost never complicated, and do not interfere with normal development. All other elements of the history and physical examination are normal, and there is nothing in the family history or genetic background to suggest underlying disorders.

On occasion, a given infant may be one of a large number of children in the family, or may be reared in circumstances which bring him into contact with a large number of individuals of school age. In today's society the nursery school and early exposure to other children have accelerated this phenomenon, even in infants of families of limited size. What occurs in these settings is the repetitive exposure to new infectious agents, i.e., new to the infant, which results in repetitive infections, again of mild character. Of course, in random distribution, any one of these infections may turn out to be serious or to herald a more systemic form of the disease, such as aseptic meningitis or viral pneumonia or bronchiolitis, but in general, these are unusual in most infants' first 2 years of life.

It is against this normal background that we must consider underlying disorders that can also lead to frequent respiratory and other types of infection. At one end of the spectrum is the child with the allergic predisposition or so-called allergic diathesis. Such an individual has a genetic proclivity towards the development of an aberrant immunologic response, which results in inflammatory lesions of the respiratory and other epithelial mucosal surfaces of a noninfectious nature. Such children, if exposed initially to foods to which they are allergic and, subsequently, to airborne inhalants, may develop inflammatory allergic rhinitis or even more extensive involvement of the respiratory tract. They may also manifest recurrent episodes of diarrhea. In some of these children, otitis media will develop, and secondary bacterial infection may result in purulent complications anywhere along the respiratory tract, including the middle ear.

In general, such infants tend to have a more frequent incidence of respiratory tract disease when contrasted with nonallergic contemporaries. They are often described by parents as having constant sniffles or stuffy nose, frequently have cough, and on occasion may be detected to wheeze or even have inspiratory stridor with minor respiratory infections. It is important to note that these infants seldom develop bacterial disease of serious magnitude, and when they do, it is usually limited to the respiratory tract and easily controllable with simple measures.

Their immunologic function, apart from the allergic antibody structure, is entirely normal, and they are capable of handling most infectious agents with an appropriate primary and secondary response. The inflammatory changes in the nasal mucosa do predispose them to repeated infections, but these infections tend to be self-limited for the most part.

At the other end of the spectrum is the individual infant who by genetic predisposition, or for reasons that are not entirely clear, is unable to mount an effective immunologic response against infectious agents. A variety of disorders have been described involving the B-cell population or antibody synthesis, the T-cell population or cell-mediated immune function, or combinations of both. In addition, disorders of complement and of white cell polymorphonuclear phagocytic function have also been described.

In each instance a specific infectious susceptibility pattern can be observed, and these children are incapable of mounting an effective response against the infectious agents usually controlled by the immune factor which they lack. Thus, in B-cell deficiencies, pyogenic infections with pneumococcus and *H. influenzae*, among others, produce serious progressive infections which, were there no effective antimicrobial therapy, could well become lethal. However, since the introduction of antimicrobials in the late 1940's, such children survive each individual episode only

to have recurrent disease, often with the same organism, further illustrating their lack of specific immunologic capacity.

The infections tend to be severe, often progressive, and frequently complicated. If inadequately treated, they may well be fatal or progress to involve more organ systems than that initially infected. Infections tend to begin and localize in the respiratory and gastrointestinal tracts but rapidly invade the bloodstream, with secondary bacteremia and distant organ involvement (e.g., meningitis, osteomyelitis, etc.). In contrast, patients with T-cell deficiency with relatively intact B-cell function tend to be susceptible to viruses, particularly DNA viruses, and to fungi. They also appear to be susceptible to some gram negative bacillary infections.

Thus these T-cell deficient individuals develop severe pneumonia with cytomegalovirus and, in the days when smallpox vaccination was widely practiced, were unable to contain this virus and developed progressive forms of the infection. They also uniformly develop oral candidiasis and may have extension of this process into the esophagus and gastrointestinal tract as well as systemically. In localized areas of the United States where other fungi are endemic, such as coccidioidomycosis in the Southwest, infections with these agents may be observed in such children.

A further group of children will have combined T-cell and B-cell deficiencies and will exhibit a broad spectrum of sensitivity ranging from the pyogenic bacteria on the one hand, to viruses, fungi and parasites on the other.

Children with complement and phagocytic disorders tend to have infections with the staphylococcus and with various other opportunistic bacteria. A particular disease pattern has been described in many of these syndromes involving the lymph nodes, liver, lungs and skin. These children seldom have dramatic overwhelming infections but rather have more indolent, chronic, recurrent episodes which are only partially controlled by their immunologic response and by antibiotic administration.

This precis of immunologic function and specific infectious susceptibility serves as a counterpoint to both the normal infant and the child with the allergic diathesis. As one can readily see, the character of the infectious episode and the infectious agent are extremely critical in differentiating between an underlying immunodeficiency and a more benign disorder or a normal "unlucky" child.

FURTHER ANALYSIS OF CASES #1 AND #2

If we now apply this background knowledge to the case histories thus far dissected, we begin to appreciate that Infant #1 probably does not have a serious underlying cause for his recurrent infectious, or seemingly infectious, episodes. Rather, a pattern very suggestive of allergic diathesis is present, in that many of his episodes were afebrile and consisted simply of an inflammatory exudate without much suggesting bacterial infection.

In contrast, Infant #2 appears to fall in our B-cell deficiency syndrome, in that he has had recurrent serious infections with pyogenic organisms, including multiple infections with the same type of organism. His history is strongly suggestive of the type of specific infectious susceptibility that children with antibody synthetic disability display.

Thus at an extremely early point in our diagnostic reasoning, we can begin to suspect that among the hypotheses from which we can choose, the correct ones in each instance appear to be suggested solely by the character of the child's history. In fact, many immunologic and infectious disease consultants can often establish such a hypothesis upon telephonic referral of such children, and they most often are correct because of the match between the history elicited and the known patterns briefly described above.

Refinements in the history are also helpful. In the first infant, upon further questioning of the parents, it was discovered that a large number of family members on both sides suffered from a variety of allergic disorders ranging from allergic rhinitis to severe asthma. Although not in itself diagnostic, such a history is very suggestive of the same process occurring in this child with compatible clinical pattern.

In the second infant the family history was less rewarding. Only a scattering of seemingly unrelated diseases was present, including several instances of collagen vascular disease (rheumatoid arthritis, systemic lupus erythematosus). However, upon persistent and detailed questioning, it was discovered that a number of early infant deaths had occurred on the maternal side of the family among male infants, usually within the first year of life. These episodes occurred sometime in the past and in distant elements of the family tree, and therefore further information was difficult to delineate. This often is the case in trying to reconstruct a family tree. It was impossible in this infant's situation to identify further the types of disease the male infants who died might have had, since their deaths occurred in remote parts of the country and no autopsies were performed in any instance.

However, the occurrence of excess deaths in male infants on the maternal side of the family is strongly suggestive of an X-linked inherited disorder. Combined with the fact that we recognize a possible B-cell deficiency in this infant's historical pattern, we are now exceedingly suspicious that the child may have an X-linked B-cell deficiency which may have been manifest in other male members of his family pedigree. Our initial tentative diagnosis becomes a bit more secure, although by no means certain, at this time.

How can we then proceed? The physical examination can be very revealing or can be noncontributory. Depending upon the degree of harm that the infections have produced on the one hand and the degree of development of the individual child on the other, we may see major manifestations suggestive of immunodeficiency, or only marginal changes that cannot be differentiated from normal. For example, in Infant #1, growth and development measurements were completely within normal limits, a not too surprising finding in view of the relatively trivial nature of his "infectious episodes." Disability in this infant was never very prolonged, and despite the long array of incidents, the majority of his infancy was spent free of symptoms.

In contrast, Infant #2 had severe, and even debilitating, infections, and it was not surprising to discover he was below the 10th percentile for weight and at the 50th percentile for height. His growth appeared to have been interfered with. Further, his social development and motor development were lagging behind what would be expected for his age. This, too, is not surprising in light of his multiple, debilitating illnesses.

Specific physical examination findings were very limited in Infant #1. His mucous membranes appeared to be boggy but really were not terribly characteristic of any specific abnormality. In fact, one was struck with the normalcy of his total physical examination. In contrast, Infant #2 appeared wan, malnourished and extremely irritable. His complexion was sallow, and despite his irritability, he appeared to be hypotonic and lethargic in his responses. His physical examination revealed respiratory distress and residual rales despite the fact that his pneumonia had been effectively treated from the standpoint of reduction in fever and toxicity. Despite a careful search, lymphoid tissue could not be identified in the posterior pharynx or at any of the usual lymph node sites. His liver was palpable, and his overall span was larger than normal, but no spleen could be palpated. His skin revealed areas of previous impetigo which had scarred, and both tympanic membranes were scarred, and the landmarks were distorted. There appeared to be an old posterolateral perforation that had sealed over.

At this point the physical examination data when added to historical information appeared clearly to indict an underlying immunodeficiency as the most likely cause for the second patient's recurring infections. The consultant was now prepared to recommend specific testing of his hypotheses in both instances, and we will digress briefly to discuss the various levels of immunologic diagnosis available to the clinician.

IMMUNOLOGIC DIAGNOSIS

As with the diagnosis of anemia and certain other disorders in childhood, there is an orderly progression available to the immunologic diagnostician. Initial screening tests can be carried out in all patients in whom the diagnosis of immunodeficiency is being considered. The value of the screening test to the patient who is not immunodeficient is that it establishes firmly for the clinician and the parents the lack of any indication for further extensive procedures or for any specific immunologic therapy, such as gamma-globulin administration.

The value of the screening procedures for the child who is immunodeficient lies in their pointing the direction in which further, more extensive and sophisticated exploration can occur. Initial screening procedures consist of probes into B- and T-cell function, into complement, into cellular integrity from both the morphologic and functional standpoints, and in general measures of homeostasis.

Thus one might wish to measure the number of B- and T-cells circulating in the peripheral blood, the presence and level of serum immunoglobulins, the number and character of circulating lymphocytes and polymorphonuclear leukocytes, the presence or absence of lymphoid and thymic tissue on chest X-ray and lateral X-ray of the neck, measurement of levels of serum complement, and a simplified functional test of white cell phagocytosis called the nitroblue tetrazolium reduction test (NBT). This preliminary battery adequately samples each of the immunologic parameters.

If T-cell dysfunction is strongly suspected, one may wish to apply appropriate skin tests based on previous clinical history (such as *Candida*, if oral moniliasis has been present) or, more precisely, submit the patient's peripheral blood to lymphocyte stimulation testing as an indirect index of normal lymphocyte function. Ordinarily, for examples of the type of disease encountered and typified by Infant #1 (the nonimmunodeficient child), this battery will suffice. One would expect all measurements to be normal except possibly for serum immunoglobulin E determination, which may be elevated. One need go no further, in that the hypothesis has basically been negated (i.e., that immunodeficiency is not present) and further tests would be futile, time-wasting and unnecessary.

In the second infant one would anticipate that the number of circulating B-cells would be reduced and that immunoglobulin levels would be low to absent. Lymphoid tissue would not be visualized in the pharynx, and all other measures of immune function will likely be normal. At this point the basic hypothesis has been verified, but sufficient delineation of the B-cell deficiency has not yet occurred. As a result, one would move on to higher levels of sophistication and specific measures of antibody capacity, of plasma cells present and immunoglobulin-staining characteristics, and other more sophisticated tests can be applied. It is beyond the scope of this chapter to discuss such issues further except simply to point out that multiple layers of refinement exist in the delineation of immunologic disorders, which are guided by each preceding step and by the clinical characteristics of the presentation.

CONCLUDING COMMENTS

We have not attempted in this analysis to cover the entire spectrum of immunologic disorders. Rather, we have tried to use two classic illustrations to indicate the degree to which diagnostic reasoning can proceed based on accurate, precise, historical data, a comprehensive physical examination, and screening laboratory tests aimed at the specific hypothesis.

However, not all patients fall neatly into the two extremes. On occasion, individuals are encountered whose histories are strongly suggestive of immunodeficiency but in whom the screening procedures are either negative or equivocal. In such instances one would press for more sophisticated determinants to sort out the many subtypes of immunodeficiency that are known to exist, impelled largely by the classic characteristics of each of the syndromes observed in a given child. On occasion, children may have an extremely suggestive history, but no immunodeficiency can be discovered despite extensive laboratory investigation. Such individuals could represent a new syndrome; in fact, many of the "old" syndromes began in just such a fashion.

Alternatively, one may have an individual whose clinical characteristics occur in a genetic setting in which the diagnosis is strongly suspected despite a limited opportunity for disease manifestation. In such instances the history may be negative, or only mild or moderate in character, and not in itself strongly suggestive of an underlying immunodeficiency. In these cases the clinician is guided mostly by the genetic circumstances which strongly suggest that the infant under consideration may be subject to the same genetic influences as previous members of his family. In such instances the screening determinations may well be abnormal prior to the occurrence of a specific disease pattern. The hypothesis that's established must be more speculative than that observed in the second infant, but it is no less sound.

As more of the syndromes are delineated and their genetic patterns uncovered, families have become increasingly suspicious that this newly born child may be subject to the same disease state. A very frequent phenomenon today is the necessity to evaluate a newly born infant for the presence of immunodeficiency before there has been any opportunity for disease expression. This is especially true in the B-cell antibody disorders, since maternally transferred immunoglobulin G will protect the infant during the first few months of life from serious disease manifestations. In these instances the hypothesis again is more speculative than in Infant #2 and may more often be answered in the negative, since most of the disorders are recessive in character and will not be expressed in every subsequent family member, even those of the same sex.

OTHER CONSIDERATIONS OF RECURRENT INFECTIONS THAT DO NOT INVOLVE SPECIFIC IMMUNODEFICIENCIES

Thus far in this chapter we have confined ourselves to exploration of the child with recurrent infections in which the character of the individual episodes and the frequency of infection suggest a generalized immunodeficiency. As we move from infancy into childhood we discover a large number of children who, upon ultimate investigation, have no specific immunodeficiency but who do suffer from repetitive infections. Examples include recurrent Group A beta-hemolytic streptococcal pharyngitis, recurrent urinary tract infections, recurrent otitis media, recurrent impetigo, and recurrent or persistent pneumonias. Many other examples could be cited, but this list will give you some idea of the flavor of this type of complaint.

In these instances our current knowledge does not permit us to understand the underlying disturbed pathophysiology. Generalized immunodeficiencies do not exist in such children, at least as measured by our present tools. If a specific immunodeficiency exists, e.g., a specific insensitivity to Group A beta-hemolytic streptococcal antibody response, we are incapable of delineating it.

In some children, mechanical factors are important, such as distortions of the eustachian tube in recurrent otitis media, or functional or anatomic disturbances in the urinary tract in chronic, recurrent urinary tract infections. Most of these children must be treated individually, their case histories carefully delineated, and all possible factors leading to the recurrent nature of their episodes explored. No simple generalization will suffice for all such instances or for all such children who experience such repetitive infections.

In some cases, epidemiologic factors, such as transmission within a family or within a specific population group, will be responsible, and in others the results of localized inflammatory disease will influence subsequent recurrences in the same anatomic site. With such diverse pathophysiologic mechanisms it is not possible to offer a specific approach to such children except to suggest that the sound principles discussed in the early chapters need to be applied vigorously in pursuit of any factor that may be uncovered. As an example of this, we will cite the occurrence of multiple streptococcal infections in a 10-year-old child.

Case #3

A 10-year-old girl had been seen repeatedly since age 5 for episodes of acute exudative tonsillopharyngitis. In each instance, Group A beta-hemolytic streptococcus was identified on throat culture, and in each instance she received multiple courses of penicillin therapy, both orally and by injection, eradicating her infection and restoring her to her usual state of good health. In the last year the physician had resorted to culturing her at a time when she was symptom-free and discovered that only occasionally did she have Group A streptococcus recoverable, and these episodes were transient in nature. The family and physician were frustrated by the multiple recurrences which frequently resulted in loss of school time and intermittent disability which distracted her from her athletic and social pursuits. They were contemplating a tonsillectomy as an attempt to end the succession of episodes of tonsillopharyngitis, and the child was referred at this point for a consultative opinion.

ANALYSIS OF CASE #3

The same principles can be applied to the delineation of this child's difficulty as have been outlined in previous chapters of a general nature. First, the data were collected carefully and thoroughly, with attention focused on possible sources of acquisition of streptococci. It appeared clear from last year's bacteriologic investigation that the child, herself, did not appear to be a chronic carrier with intermittent flaring of acute episodes, as has occasionally been described. Attention, therefore, was turned to her epidemiologic groups in order to discover external contacts which might be reinfecting her with the Group A streptococcus. The most immediate group that was considered was her immediate family and family-like contacts.

It was discovered that on occasion other members of the family had experienced Group A beta-hemolytic streptococcal infections but with nowhere near the frequency that our 10-year-old patient had. However, when these infections were plotted over time, it was clear that the family appeared to keep the streptococcus alive within its midst, with various members experiencing overt disease at random and with this child experiencing overt disease consistently.

A further search did not reveal any similar patterns in her school-age companions or in the close-knit Sunday school group that she attended at her church.

Laboratory determinations were not extensive in this child, since previous investigators have clearly demonstrated that no specific immunologic deficiency exists among such children, and that such a search would be futile. Apart from reculturing her at a time when she was asymptomatic to ascertain again whether or not she carried streptococcus and to determine her antibody responses to the various enzymes of the streptococcus, nothing further was done at that point. However, it was recommended that with the child's next episode the entire family be cultured and, from that point on, any streptococci isolated be considered infectious and the family member from whom the streptococcus was isolated be treated simultaneously with this child.

Over the course of the next 6 months it was clearly determined that infections tended to ping-pong in the family, and that prompt therapy of all positive family members resulted in fewer episodes at longer intervals. Eventually this young lady had only intermittent infections which were easily controllable when the entire family was viewed as a single epidemiologic unit.

This success story should not lull us into believing that all such episodes end so benignly. In another family that the author has treated in the past, ping-ponging occurred despite simultaneous treatment of all family members at the time the index case experienced the next episode of streptococcal tonsillopharyngitis. Despite application of the therapeutic regimen outlined above, no real impact was made upon this family, and ultimately, monthly doses of benzathine penicillin were prescribed for all family members for a period of 3 months, during which no infections were experienced. Upon removal of such therapy the same ping-ponging pattern recurred and could not be prevented.

I could easily have cited examples of urinary tract infection or recurrent pneumonia to illustrate typical underlying pathologic processes in these very different infections. However, such consideration would lead to excessive repetition. The principles are unvarying, the specific episodes myriad. By understanding the process, one can apply it to specific instances almost irrespective of content. Of course, specific knowledge in each area is essential.

Chapter 13

The Child with Diarrhea

INTRODUCTION

The diagnostic challenge presented by a child with a diarrheal illness is a complex one. Simultaneously with consideration of etiology, the physician must also assess fluid and electrolyte balance, central nervous system morphologic and functional status, cardiovascular function and renal capacity. Also, the clinician must decide if the diarrheal symptoms are the primary problem or just one part of a more diffuse infection. Thus, what appears to be a simple decision-making process really consists of several decisions.

In individual children the priority given to the assessments listed above will differ. For example, the febrile child with mild diarrheal illness and no other symptoms will direct the physician to homeostatic assessment first. Etiologic evaluation will only briefly be considered in deference to the more critical determination of how disturbed the child's fluid and electrolyte balance has become. On the other hand, if a child presents with fever, grand mal seizure, and shock with diarrhea, the etiologic agent and the disturbance of homeostasis achieve similar importance in the diagnostic process. It is true that even in this circumstance, homeostasis must first be assessed and the disturbances managed, but consideration of etiology must occur in order to apply prompt and correct therapy.

HOMEOSTATIC ANALYSIS

The physician must make a rapid clinical assessment of the following factors in a child with diarrhea:

1. fluid loss
2. electrolyte imbalance
3. state of hydration
4. extracellular volume status

Fluid loss can be gauged by historical clues—the duration of the diarrhea, the number and character of the stools, the degree of fever (increased insensitive water loss), the fluid intake during the period of loss, and the presence or absence of vomiting. All of these factors contribute to an educated guess as to whether the loss has been severe, moderate or mild in extent. Further refinement can be achieved by attention to the frequency of urination (decrease implies fluid conservation or dysfunctional bladder or both), the presence or absence of tears (indicative of degree of dehydration), and the continuation and pace of losses from the gastrointestinal (GI) tract.

The clinician establishes a homeostatic "guess" based on such details which places the patient on a scale from little fluid loss to severe loss. Even further refinement occurs as a result of physical examination, but since diarrhea is a common and often mild disease, the described historical points may suffice. In such situations the clinician may prescribe methods to decrease loss (such as no further feeding or significant alteration in the content of ingested foods or fluids) and to replace previously incurred losses. This is often done without the need for physical examination and based solely upon telephonic data collection. In this instance the diagnostic reasoning involves a decision that implies a nontreatable, nonserious etiologic cause plus a judgement that homeostasis has not been greatly disturbed. Implicit to this line of reasoning are the known facts, that such instances of diarrhea are self-limited and that the fluid loss is easily correctable with oral replacement.

The accuracy of such reasoning is gauged by the infant or child's response to the recommended oral rehydration. This is usually assessed by continuous telephonic communication which regauges the criteria discussed above.

In contrast, initial historic data may yield the judgement that the fluid loss has been excessive and that simple measures for control will not suffice. If the history is that of profuse water loss stools, of inadequate urination, of lack of tears, of change in alertness, of vomiting, or of combinations of these, the physician will be alerted to the necessity for physical evaluation of the child. Historical features such as those described above will usually mandate that the child be evaluated personally by the physician.

Physical assessment will focus on observation of the actual character of the stool, on the vital signs in the infant, on the state of hydration, and on specific evidence of disturbances in other systems. These data add a degree of precision to the historical information and lead to a decision as to the need for other than oral replacement therapy and to the urgency of instituting such replacement.

Severe disturbances in homeostasis are suggested by positive historical data confirmed by the presence of certain changes on the physical examination of the infant. Hypotension, severely depressed affect or frank coma, 15% or greater dehydration, or shock are the most serious findings in a spectrum of changes that are determinable by physical examination data.

Thus the physician will use the progressive assessment of historical and physical examination data to determine the degree of homeostatic disturbance and the need for specific testing of such disturbance.

ELECTROLYTE IMBALANCE

Most diarrheal illness involves isotonic loss of electrolytes. The stool in these instances contains concentrations of sodium and other electrolytes at approximately the same level as that found in plasma. In mild diarrheal illness no attempt is made to assess with accuracy the exact changes in electrolyte composition. The clinician again relies upon the self-limiting character of the disease and the fact that normal renal function will correct and adjust minor aberrations in electrolyte concentration, given adequate blood flow and an appropriate ingestion of an isotonic fluid. In these instances, "nature" is heavily relied upon to provide the mechanisms for preservation of homeostasis.

In contrast, some infants will excrete larger concentrations of electrolyte in relation to water than that found in plasma. They will develop hypoelectrolytemic dehydration. Minor degrees of hypoelectrolytemia are undetectable clinically and can only be assayed by analysis of plasma electrolyte concentration. In many instances, minor deviations in mild diarrhea will go undetected and be corrected in the process of oral rehydration and adequate renal function.

Severe hyponatremia (a sodium concentration equal to or less than 120 mEq/liter) is usually accompanied by detectable signs and symptoms. If the reduction in sodium concentration has been gradual, the child will exhibit increasing apathy, increasing anorexia, nausea, vomiting and some mental confusion. A sudden loss resulting in hyponatremic plasma levels may result in severe headache, coma or severe mental impairment, delirium, and some muscular dysfunction. If the levels are sustained, generalized convulsions may occur. The central nervous system signs described are attributable to hypoosmolarity which results in intracellular accumulation of water in the brain. This is the so-called water intoxication syndrome.

A specific subset of hyponatremic infants develop this state secondary to inappropriate secretion of antidiuretic hormone (IADH) (vasopressin). This IADH syndrome is referred to as "inappropriate" because it occurs despite a normal extracellular fluid volume.

Uncommon in primary diarrheal states the IADH syndrome can occur with many other disorders in which diarrhea is a component (e.g., meningitis, pneumonia, etc.).

At the other end of the electrolyte-loss spectrum, hyperelectrolytemia occurs because water loss is more than electrolyte loss. Most commonly, in diarrheal disease, it results from replacement by hyperosmolar fluids in the face of continued water loss. The infant may initially experience isotonic diarrhea, but if a high solute-containing fluid, such as milk, is offered and accepted, the child may accumulate electrolyte in the plasma. If errors are made in oral replacement solutions which result in a high sodium concentration being offered the infant, the development of hyperelectrolytemia may be enhanced. In infants who are losing more water than electrolyte, even isotonic replacement may result in hyperelectrolytemia. In a few infants, excessive fever of prolonged duration may result in a heightened insensible water loss. These infants are prone to develop hyperelectrolytemia on the basis of this excessive loss.

Hyperelectrolytemia is suggested clinically if the history reveals a high solute or hyperosmolar oral replacement, or prolonged or high fever, or if the physical examination fails to demonstrate a degree of dehydration which is consistent with the extent of fluid loss by history. The latter finding occurs secondary to intracellular accumulation of water, and leads to the finding of normal or near-normal skin turgor and a "doughy" feel to the skin, fat and subcutaneous tissues. Such infants may even proceed to shock without significant external evidence of dehydration. Additional historical clues include irritability, stupor or coma, irregular respirations, and convulsions. In addition, lack of sweating, either by history or by observation, and excessive thirst may be detected in some children.

Specific electrolyte dysfunctions occur in some diarrheal states. However, for the most part, losses of electrolytes are uniform, and single component disturbances are more often related to inadequate replacement than to a specific loss or retention. However, some children with shigellosis may exhibit profound hypotonia secondary to marked potassium depletion. This appears to occur as a result of the primary infection but is often aggravated by inadequate or late replacement of potassium in oral or intravenous fluids.

In malabsorbent diarrheas, loss of calcium and magnesium may be severe, as soaps are formed by these cations with fatty acids in the stool. Clinical signs include muscle weakness and wasting, irritability, and signs of neuromuscular junction dysfunction (Chvostek's sign, tremors, fasciculations and convulsions).

In addition to the electrolyte imbalance disturbances, acid base metabolism may be altered. Most often, metabolic acidosis accompanies acute infectious diarrhea. Loss of buffer base results in a lowering of the pH which is aggravated by accumulation of nonvolatile organic acids. Base excess values may reach very low levels and are clinically detectable as hyperventilation.

Rarely, in diarrheal states in which vomiting is severe, loss of excessive amounts of acid may result in metabolic alkalosis overwhelming the metabolic acidosis which is secondary to the diarrhea. Also, chronic diarrhea with loss of chloride may produce alkalosis.

ASSESSMENT OF DEHYDRATION

The principal effect of diarrhea is loss of body fluids in excess of ingested replacement. The result is dehydration with fluid shifts between the various body compartments. The most disastrous result is sufficient loss of intravascular volume to produce shock. A continuous spectrum of loss may be encountered short of shock.

In general, the use of the rule of 5's is employed in assessing dehydration. Mild dehydration is considered to be at the 5% or less body weight loss level, severe dehydration at the 10% level, and shock at the 15% level. This convenient clinical guide is only an approximation but is useful. If it is employed, one must remember that it is an approximation and is based upon isotonic or hypotonic dehydration and is not applicable in hyperelectrolytemia (at least as far as clinical clues are concerned).

In the rule of 5 system, one uses the degree

of change in skin turgor, in the dehydration of the periorbital tissues, and in the state of the fontanel to gauge the degree. It is best to use actual body weight, when available, but in most clinical situations, accurate prediarrheal weight determination is seldom available.

At 5% dehydration the skin turgor is poor, but the disturbed skin will return to its normal contour in a few seconds, the eyes are not sunken, and the fontanel is flat. At 10% dehydration the skin turgor is poor and the disturbed skin remains tented, often for minutes after disturbance, and the eyes and fontanel are sunken, but shock is not present. At 15% dehydration all of the features of 10% dehydration are present and marked, and blood pressure is depressed.

The usefulness of these criteria is found in therapeutic decision making. At 5% dehydration or less, most infants can be managed with oral replacement, most often as outpatients. At 10% dehydration, hospitalization and intravenous replacement are mandatory. Of course, at 15% dehydration, urgent measures to counteract shock are employed. Between 5 and 10% dehydration an individual assessment must be made relying on family and social factors as much as on actual degree and pace of loss.

ETIOLOGIC ASSESSMENT

Given the homeostatic state of a given infant, etiologic diagnosis is also critical to determine the need for hospitalization and for therapeutic and public health management. Usually the critical decision sought is whether or not a treatable cause of the diarrhea is present.

The vast majority of infantile and early childhood diarrhea is due to viral infection of the GI tract alone or as part of a more generalized viral infection. It is now possible to identify specific viral agents responsible for diarrhea, although this is not attempted in all instances. It reguires an electron microscopic examination of the stool for rotovirus or standard viral isolation techniques for other agents responsible for diarrhea. The clinician usually relies upon the characteristic clinical features of viral diarrhea and on oc-

casion will use nonspecific and specific laboratory tests to rule out bacterial and other causes.

Viral diarrhea is characterized by smallbowel dysfunction in which water and electrolyte absorption by surface cells is impaired, resulting in net loss of water to the body. There is little or no obvious inflammatory component. Thus, water loss stools are produced and GI motility is increased. The child has frequent, large watery stools. For example, the diaper may have little fecal content but will be soaked with water. Fever is usually absent or minimal, and abdominal pain absent or mild. Vomiting is frequent but usually not severe. Convulsions and other systemic symptoms and signs are usually absent.

Examination of the stool confirms the pathophysiology of viral gastroenteritis. There are no inflammatory cells, and there is no blood or mucus. The stool is usually odorless.

Unfortunately, toxic diarrheas may have similar characteristics. The toxin may be of endogenous origin (bacteria such as *Escherichia coli* or the vibrios) or of exogenous origin (food poisoning syndromes, for example). One difference in toxic diarrheas is the usual presence of mucus, occasionally in abundance.

Also, giardiasis may produce a similar diarrheal pattern. *Giardia lamblia* finds residence in the small bowel and somehow alters intestinal absorption, leading to water loss stools. It also causes a temporary lactase deficiency which further aggravates water loss by osmotic effect. The only discernible difference in pattern from viral diarrhea is that which, caused by *Giardia*, may not be self-limited, and a continuous or intermittent disease may result.

In contrast to viral, toxic and giardial disease, invasive bacteria and parasites produce dysenteric syndromes marked by inflammatory changes in the bowel. The diarrhea produced is viscous, and the stool is filled with inflammatory cells, destroyed and shed intestinal epithelial cells, and blood. The stool may be odorless or have a musty to foul odor. Mucus is almost always present, often in abundance. The inflammatory disease results in intestinal contractions and intermittent, crampy abdominal pain, often severe. Tenesmus, or pain on defecation, also occurs. Vomiting is variable.

Some invasive bacterial diarrheal states have characteristic features. In shigellosis a convulsion may precede or accompany the first abnormal stool. The anal sphincter tone tends to be lax in *Shigella* infections. In *Salmonella* dysentery the stool may be foulsmelling, and bacteremia may occur, particularly in young infants. In *Campylobacter* dysentery, severe abdominal pain and fever may precede or accompany profuse watery diarrhea with blood.

Amebiasis will occur with sufficient frequency in some areas of the country to enter the differential diagnosis. Amebiasis may resemble the dysenteric states described above. The stool almost always contains blood; most often gross blood is found, but occasionally it can only be detected microscopically. There are no white blood cells in the stool, a distinguishing feature from invasive bacterial dysentery.

RELATIONSHIP OF DIARRHEA TO OTHER ILLNESSES

Thus far we have only considered diarrhea occurring as a primary entity, e.g., acute infectious gastroenteritis. It is clear that not all instances of diarrhea fall into this category. Acute diarrhea can occur in the following instances:

1. as part of an infection other than in the GI tract (so-called parenteral diarrhea)
2. as a result of malnutrition
3. as part of a metabolic or endocrine disease pattern (e.g., hyperthyroidism)
4. secondary to mechanical and/or structural disease of the GI tract
5. as a result of dietary abnormalities
6. secondary to drugs, especially antibiotics
7. due to allergic disorders
8. secondary to malabsorptive disorders
9. as the first episode in a more chronic diarrheal state (e.g., intractable diarrhea of infancy, regional enteritis)
10. due to miscellaneous causes

It is not the purpose of this chapter to explore each of these categories in detail. It should be evident from examination of the above list that a complete data base is necessary for any of these conditions to be considered as possible hypotheses in an individual case. Such historical clues as mode of onset, association with changes in diet, association with drug ingestion, association with other symptoms, and the specifics of the epidemiology of a given patient's illness can all lead to suspicions that a cause other than acute infection is present.

The physical examination can be critical. Detection of the focus of infection other than in the GI tract, the presence of evidence of malnutrition, the presence of signs of metabolic or endocrine disorders, and the specific findings on the abdominal examination—all may contribute to diagnostic delineation of the problem.

PUTTING IT ALL TOGETHER

The child with acute diarrheal illness thus poses a specific set of reasoning problems for the diagnostician. Initial historical assessment can usually establish the degree of disability anticipated and will provide potential clues to the etiology of the diarrhea. A judgement must be made as to the adequacy of the history alone as a guide for hypothesis setting and for clinical action. In these instances the clinician recognizes that his data base is incomplete and that his hypotheses are speculative and untested, and he relies upon the subsequent clinical sequence to determine the correctness of his assumptions.

If the history is suggestive of a severity greater than a "mild" categorization, the physical examination data become critical. Completion of physical assessment may again be sufficient to make hypotheses which do not require testing other than by subsequent clinical sequence. This may result in the clinician taking clinical action and establishing rehydration of the infant or child without the intervening necessity for obtaining laboratory determinations.

Alternatively, the clinician may decide that tests of homeostasis or etiology or both are mandatory. At this point he must evoke economical considerations—economy being defined both in terms of financial cost and in terms of convenience and necessity.

In moderate diarrhea of presumptive viral etiology he may choose simply to verify the degree of hydration and electrolyte imbalance without further test of etiology. To do so, a hemoglobin and hematocrit level, urinalysis, and serum electrolyte and pH determinations may suffice. The degree of hemoconcentration, the level of the blood urea nitrogen, and the specific gravity of the urine will serve as an assessment of the state of hydration. The electrolyte concentrations will place the disorder in the appropriate category, and the pH level will gauge the presence and degree of acidosis.

For further refinement, stool examination for virus particles is available.

In severe diarrheal disease the physician may add blood gas determination, electrocardiographic assessment (for disturbances of potassium) and more specific etiologic determinations, such as examination of the stools for white blood cells and by culture.

In instances of a dysenteric pattern to the diarrhea, tests will be utilized to identify the various bacterial agents and, if suspected, *G. lamblia* and ameba.

Thus one can see a progression of diagnostic reasoning, hypothesis setting, and laboratory testing. It is not a willy-nilly "everything and everybody" pattern. Rather, diagnostic tests are predicated on clinical reasoning and on presumptive homeostatic and etiologic hypotheses.

Similarly, clinical reasoning and decisions as to therapy also rely on a progressive analysis backed up by specific tests. The decisions range from simple oral rehydration to emergent antishock therapy, and from no specific therapy through nonspecific symptomatic relief measures to specific antimicrobial treatment. These various actions are dependent upon logical thought and well-conceived hypotheses which have been adequately tested. Although the content differs from other problems commented upon in this volume, the process does not.

Chapter 14

The Child with Inspiratory Stridor or Expiratory Wheezing

INTRODUCTION

A child's inability to breathe without difficulty generates a great deal of anxiety for parents and medical caretakers alike. Interruption to the free flow of air from its ingress at the mouth and nose to its ultimate distant destination in the alveoli, and from the reverse route it travels, will most often result in noises that can be perceived by the naked ear or with a stethoscope. Such noises are symptomatic of structural and physiologic disturbances in the normal lumen of the airway. If the sound produced is on inhalation and results from disturbance in laminar flow secondary to a narrowed lumen in the upper airway, the sound produced is called stridor.

If, on the other hand, the impediment to free laminar flow is in the expiratory phase and takes place in the lower airways, the sound produced is called wheezing. Unfortunately, most parents and some physicians do not distinguish between these two quite different sounds and refer to both as wheezing. Since the pathophysiologic significance differs markedly between the two types of turbulent air flow, it is critical for the clinician to carefully define whether stridor, or wheezing, or both are present, as defined above. This is not an academic matter, as both diagnostic and therapeutic decisions will be based upon the precise pathophysiologic disturbance. Misunderstanding of the underlying pathophysiology, and misinterpretation of sounds produced in the obstructed airway, have resulted in inappropriate therapy for specific conditions and in delays in appropriate diagnostic tests for obstructive lesions.

Inspiratory stridor is created because of turbulent air flow past a point of obstruction. In general, the obstruction is at the supralaryngeal to subglottic levels. The obstruction may be mechanical, inflammatory, or a combination of both. As we will shortly consider, the specific etiologic differential diagnosis will be dependent initially upon precise definition of the most likely site of origin of the perceived sound. In contrast, expiratory wheezing is most often best appreciated with a stethoscope and occurs because of obstruction at the prealveolar level.

In some clinical circumstances a more gross type of wheezing is produced which is audible to the naked ear. This gross expiratory sound may be produced because of a narrowed lumen in the larger branches of the tracheobronchial tree or because of mucus, pus or other material within the lumen. On some occasions, the noise perceived is both an inspiratory gurgle and an expiratory wheeze secondary to these same factors. This spectrum of sounds, from inspiratory stridor to expiratory wheezing, has led to considerable confusion among the laity, and to some extent among professionals, as to the precise meaning of wheezing.

In this chapter we will discuss the diagnostic approach to the child who has the acute onset of noisy respirations, as defined above.

CASE HISTORIES

Case #1

A 4-year-old child is brought to the emergency room because earlier in the day he developed a temperature of 104° F and complained of inability to swallow because of pain. The parents also felt that his voice had changed and become more "distant." Just prior to bringing him to your attention, he began to have difficulty breathing, and the parents described hearing a wheezing sound as if he were "struggling to get air in." On physical examination you see an anxious, markedly flushed 4-year-old who has saliva drooling from the corners of his mouth. He is holding his hand on his neck as if in great discomfort. With each inspiration there is a loud, high-pitched sighing sound. His temperature is 105° F, his pulse rate is 160/min, and his respiratory rate is 30/min. Rapid stethoscopic examination reveals the same sound as is audible without the stethoscope, heard best with the stethoscope placed over the neck. The rest of his chest examination is clear.

Case #2

A 6-year-old boy became ill earlier in the day with fever to 104° F, lassitude and anorexia. He had had a mild upper respiratory tract infection for the past 2 days without fever and without much change in his physical activity or appetite. In the last 2 hours the parents have noticed that he is breathing more rapidly and appears to be wheezing and "struggling to catch his breath." Since this latter symptom had become worse, they decided to bring him to your office.

On physical examination his temperature is 103° F, his pulse rate is 160/min, and his respiratory rate is 40/min. He appears listless and has a marked mucoid discharge running from both nostrils. When first seen, he is holding on to the back of a chair and appears to be exerting maximum effort at breathing. A rapid stethoscopic examination reveals multiple, high-pitched squeaking sounds on expiration scattered throughout his entire thorax.

CASE ANALYSIS

These two children represent quite different pathophysiologic processes, although superficially they resemble each other. Both are febrile, both are in marked distress, and both have breathing difficulty. In the first instance the child's onset was acute, and the complaints preceding respiratory difficulty were those of a sore throat and difficulty on swallowing. In the second child, respiratory inflammatory disease had been present for some time prior to the development of fever and respiratory difficulty. There was no historical evidence of pain on swallowing or breathing. Both children are seriously ill and exerting maximum effort in respiration. If, for the moment, one leaves all other symptoms aside and considers only the examination of the respiratory tract, the difference between the two boys becomes apparent. In the first child the difficulty is on inspiration, and his respiratory effort is to breathe air in and appears localized to the upper airway with no physical findings related to his lungs. In the second child the difficulty is almost totally related to inability to expire. Air entry seems unimpaired despite the rapidity of respirations. His difficulty is in smoothly removing air from the distal parts of his lung.

These two extreme examples illustrate dramatically the difference between inspiratory stridor and expiratory wheezing. In the first instance the child was subsequently determined to have *Hemophilus influenzae* epiglottitis, an inflammatory disease limited to the upper airway and involving inflammatory edema of the epiglottis, the aryepiglottic folds and the larynx. The resultant effect is to narrow the airway at the point of entry into the tracheobronchial tree. Inspiratory stridor occurs because the air must now enter the lungs through a greatly narrowed opening, and the turbulent, rapid flow produces the sound we call stridor.

In the second child, air entry is free. However, once it reaches the alveoli it cannot easily be released by passive effort. Upon more detailed history it was discovered that this child had had episodes of asthma in the past. This episode was bronchial asthma complicating an upper respiratory tract infection, probably of viral origin. His pathophysiologic lesion was edema and bronchoconstriction of the terminal bronchioles resulting in a narrowed lumen which on expiration resulted in turbulent and rapid air flow, resulting in the characteristic squeaking sound we call expiratory wheezing.

Within minutes the experienced clinician will distinguish these two syndromes and be directed in two quite different diagnostic and therapeutic endeavors. In the first instance he will attempt to establish immediately an airway to bypass the increasing obstructive lesion which, if untended, can and does result in total respiratory obstruction and cardiovascular collapse. The child may die with a totally obstructed upper airway. In the second instance, attention will be directed toward the relief of bronchospasm, which is the major component of the obstruction. After immediate relief, the physician will then consider the etiologic role of the upper respiratory tract infection and other environmental factors which have resulted in this particular episode of expiratory obstruction termed asthma.

These two cases dramatically illustrate the absolute need for precise data collection and delineation prior to attempting any therapy. Had the clinician mistakenly interpreted the first child's illness for a more generalized respiratory infection, he may have delayed appropriate establishment of an airway, which may have had lethal consequences. In the second instance it was necessary to perceive the level of obstruction as distal in the tracheobronchial tree in order to direct therapeutic attention to its correction and to avoid unnecessary diagnostic exploration of the rest of the respiratory system. These two instances are rather obvious and were chosen because they best illustrate the extremes.

There are children who will develop an upper respiratory tract infection and have both inspiratory stridor and some evidence of lower respiratory tract lesions. In some instances, children will present with a typical croup-like syndrome, with inspiratory stridor, an upper respiratory tract infection, and both rales and wheezing upon examination of the chest. We have come to appreciate that many instances of so-called croup in fact are generalized respiratory tract infections in which the more predominant feature is upper airway obstruction but by no means is the exclusive lesion.

Thus the first step in the approach to the child with stridor or wheezing is to define accurately which of the two is present or, if both are present, which is predominant.

ETIOLOGIC CAUSES OF INSPIRATORY STRIDOR

Before we further consider the diagnostic approach to the child with stridor, once we have established that that is the primary clinical presentation, we must consider the range of possibilities. Acute inspiratory stridor is due to mechanical or inflammatory causes or a combination of these.

Mechanical causes can occur without inflammatory changes. A child may obstruct a portion of the upper airway by inhalation of a foreign body. The ingress of air is obstructed by the presence of the body in the lumen of the airway, and inspiratory stridor can result. Apart from this type of obstruction, most mechanical lesions of the upper airway become evident because of the addition of an inflammatory component. Thus the child who has an obstructive lesion of minimal degree, based on a congenital anomaly or the like, may only manifest stridor if an upper respiratory tract infection supervenes.

Among the predisposing causes of a mechanical nature are anomalies of the epiglottis and aryepiglottic folds, congenital webs and narrowings of the larynx and subglottic areas, and subglottic masses of both benign and malignant nature. This type of lesion may be present for long periods of time without producing significant clinical symptomatology. With the onset of an acute upper respiratory tract infection, sufficient edema is added to the initial obstructing lesion to narrow the airway further to the point at which inspiratory stridor is produced.

In some children, no mechanical precursor is necessary for an inflammatory disease to produce sufficient edema to obstruct the upper airway. The classical illness that produces inspiratory stridor, primarily because of an inflammatory component, is viral croup. Alternatively termed laryngotracheobronchitis, croup is a disease in which inflammation of the airway is accentuated in the larynx or subglottic areas with subsequent obstruction. Most often, croup is due to an acute viral infection. However, there are some children whose croup syndrome is repeatedly manifest, and these instances have been thought due to an allergic disorder or to another undefined reason for irritability of the upper airway. In either instance, the result clinically is the same. The child presents repeatedly with respiratory stridor of acute onset.

As illustrated in Case #1 above, bacterial infection of the upper airway may also produce inspiratory stridor. The classic example here is *H. influenzae* epiglottitis. In this lesion the inflammation is localized to the epiglottis and aryepiglottic folds. The inflammation itself may be more extensive, and most often is, as many of these children are bacteremic and some have evidence of more extensive respiratory disease. However, the predominant feature is obstruction of the upper airway, and it is this component of the infection that is most often lethal.

On rare occations a more distal obstructing lesion may be present and become evident as an inspiratory obstructive episode. For example, anomalies of the great vessels, including a double aortic arch or anomalous intrathoracic arteries, may sufficiently impinge upon the trachea to produce the potential for obstruction. In some instances these children will have chronic obstructive findings, but more commonly the obstruction becomes evident when an inflammatory episode supervenes.

A disputed group of lesions is thought by some to produce airway obstruction. The so-called chondromalacias supposedly involve defects in cartilage of the larynx and trachea, allowing these structures to collapse on inspiration, producing relative inspiratory insufficiency. On the other hand, some experts feel that such lesions do not exist, and that if chondromalacia is a true entity, it is extremely rare.

Uncommonly, mass lesions in and around the subglottic area will produce obstruction. Such lesions as subglottic hemangiomas, fibromas, and rare solid tumors can sufficiently impinge on the airway to produce inspiratory obstruction.

Also, tracheal abnormalities of congenital and acquired nature can lead to upper airway obstruction. Tracheostenosis has been seen occasionally as an apparently congenital event. In other children it appears to be acquired because of some insult to the trachea, such as prior intubation or a previously repaired tracheoesophageal fistula. In the latter instance, it is uncertain whether the tracheoesophageal fistula is accompanied by primary abnormalities in the trachea or whether the necessary surgical repair results in subsequent stenosis.

Of recent interest are children who occasionally present with what appears to be upper airway obstruction, and the usual causes are not found. Some of these children have been demonstrated to have gastroesophageal reflux, a condition which permits the corrosive gastric acids to enter the esophagus and produce inflammatory changes there. In some children the reflux gastric contents are aspirated and can produce tracheal changes resulting in this syndrome. More commonly, these children have recurrent pneumonia as the heralding clinical sign of gastroesophageal reflux.

Finally, there are some children who will display inspiratory stridor and despite extensive study, no etiology is found. In this group of children the reason for inspiratory stridor in unclear.

ETIOLOGY OF EXPIRATORY WHEEZING

In infancy the most common cause of expiratory wheezing is viral infection of the lower respiratory tract, most commonly with respiratory syncytial virus. This syndrome is termed bronchiolitis, and the expiratory wheezing occurs as a result of inflammatory changes in the terminal bronchioles. Although bronchospasm may be a small element in obstruction, it almost never is predominant, and it is mucosal edema and inflammation that result in the obstruction to expiration. A subset of such infants appear destined to develop asthma in later life. At the present time it is not possible to distinguish with ease those children who have a single acute episode of bronchiolitis and those who will develop recurrent episodes of wheezing that eventually will be termed bronchial asthma.

The second most common cause of expiratory wheezing is allergic asthma. Although a few children appear to have the onset in infancy, most instances of allergic asthma become evident in later childhood. Typically the child has had other allergic manifestations prior to the onset of asthma. Many different factors will trigger bronchospasm that results in expiratory wheezing and asthma. They range from infections to inhaled allergens to physical agents and to unknown factors in the environment. Common to all such instances is an airway which is hyperreactive, and the resultant bronchospasm produces expiratory wheezing.

Some children with infectious pneumonia will also have wheezing as one component of their physical examination. In these children the primary lesion is alveolar exudation with inflammatory cells and detritus. However, there may be sufficient inflammation in the terminal bronchioles to produce a bronchospastic component. Thus the rales that are heard, which are secondary to the fluid in the airway, may be accompanied by expiratory wheezes which are a direct result of bronchospasm plus edema of the bronchiolar mucosa.

Other noninfectious causes of inspiratory wheezing include chemical and specific allergic bronchiolar irritation. For example, some children after inhalation of volatile hydrocarbons will develop a severe bronchitis and pneumonia, one component of which will be bronchiolar obstruction. Similarly, there is a specific allergy to aspergillosis, an ubiquitous fungus. In these children, exposure to the fungal antigens results in intense bronchospasm, mimicking allergic asthma.

Rarely, obstructive lesions impinging on the smaller bronchi may result in an audible wheeze. For example, tuberculous nodes may compress a portion of the tracheobronchial tree, leading to an audible wheeze at the point of compression. In some instances the compressing lesion may erode into the bronchus, leading to endobronchial disease which also can produce expiratory wheezing.

A few hereditary diseases may result in episodes of expiratory wheezing. Cystic fibrosis and alpha$_1$-antitrypsin deficiency may have sufficient pulmonary manifestations to produce pneumonic changes, one component of which may be bronchiolar restriction.

The above descriptions of the etiology and mechanisms of expiratory stridor and expiratory wheezing are not meant to be totally inclusive. Other conditions not mentioned above can produce either or both lesions on rare occasions. Their exclusion is not critical to our subsequent analysis.

FURTHER ANALYSIS OF THE CHILD WITH STRIDOR OR WHEEZING

Having established the anatomic localization responsible for the audible sounds produced by obstructed respiration, we can now turn our attention to the further diagnostic analysis of the individual child's problem. We must keep in mind the possible etiologic categories responsible for each of the syndromes.

In conditions with inspiratory stridor as the predominant manifestation, the primary consideration facing the physician is how quickly he must act. Thus the initial decision is a homeostatic one, the purpose of which is to sustain life by sustaining an adequate airway and adequate oxygenation. In all instances of inspiratory obstruction at the upper airway level, the clinician must first consider the degree to which the child's life is threatened. Various factors are utilized in making such a judgement. The first is the knowledge of the usual way in which the lesions that are life-threatening present. One must know that epiglottitis can result in rapid closure of the airway and in death within hours of onset. One must further appreciate that most viral croup will not be life-threatening, but that in a few instances, sufficient obstruction occurs that the lesion is as lethal as that seen in epiglottitis. Similarly, one must recognize that an inhaled foreign body, if of sufficient size and if accompanied by marked laryngospasm, may also be life-threatening. In short, there is no substitute for adequate knowledge of each of the major entities that produce inspiratory obstruction. Thus, on the initial assessment, the clinician asks the question,

"Is this lesion obstructing the airway in such fashion that the child's life is in jeopardy?"

To answer this question the clinician initially utilizes clinical assessment. Historical information of importance is whether or not the lesion was of sudden onset and whether or not it was accompanied by other manifestations. For example, in *H. influenzae* epiglottitis the disease almost always is abrupt in onset and heralded by dysphagia and changes in the tone of the voice. Sudden high fever is also characteristic. In viral croup the onset tends to be insidious, often preceded by one or more days of an upper respiratory infection. In other forms of croup the onset may be more abrupt, particularly if a preexisting lesion which partially obstructed the airway is enhanced by inflammatory edema. If the onset of inspiratory stridor was abrupt in a nonfebrile child, the question of an inhaled foreign body must be considered, and the circumstances under which the child developed stridor may be critical. If he had been eating peanuts or popcorn, had had a foreign object in his mouth prior to the onset, or a like history, the possibility of an inhaled foreign body must be seriously considered. Such information should be sought if the circumstances suggest an abrupt onset without preceding or accompanying upper airway inflammatory disease.

If the initial history does not suggest an emergent problem, such as epiglottitis or an inhaled foreign body, the prior history becomes critical in assessment. Was the child ill for several days prior to the onset of stridor? Is this the first episode that the child has experienced? Have there been any signs suggesting partial obstruction in the past? Are there associated congenital anomalies that suggest a congenital anomaly within the tracheobronchial tree? Etc.

The next level of assessment is by physical examination. In this instance it must be remembered that an upper airway that is already compromised may be shut off completely by diagnostic maneuvers. This is particularly true in *H. influenzae* epiglottitis, but it may also occur with other inflammatory and noninflammatory lesions. For this reason most clinicians will not undertake the examination of the upper airway in a child with

marked acute inspiratory stridor unless they are in circumstances in which immediate intubation or tracheostomy can be performed.

Alternatively, if the history and physical examination do not suggest the need for immediate intubation, the clinician may choose to examine the upper airway roentgenologically. In these circumstances the air-filled larynx and trachea provide their own contrast, and one can visualize an obstructing epiglottis (the so-called thumb sign), or alternatively, narrowed segments of the airway may be detected. This noninvasive approach has the virtue of not inducing additional laryngospasm. It has the potential disadvantage of delaying definitive therapy and must only be undertaken in situations in which complete preparation for immediate intubation is available should the delay be accompanied by progression in inspiratory obstruction. A considerable degree of experience is required to determine if roentgenologic studies are safe to proceed with. If time permits, the less experienced clinician should seek the advice and counsel and assistance of individuals more experienced with upper airway obstruction.

Additional features that can assist in the determination of the urgency of the problem in an individual child include the degree of oxygenation, the extent of respiratory effort, the degree to which fatigue in the child is interfering with respiratory effort, and the rapidity of progression while the child is under observation. Assessment needs to be calm, although rapid. At any point in the assessment process the individual must be prepared to interfere with the obstructing process and to establish a patent airway.

If we assume that immediate intervention is not necessary and that oxygenation and respiratory effort are within acceptable limits, the clinician has time to explore etiologic possibilities and to institute appropriate pharmacologic and physiologic therapy. It is beyond the scope of this text to detail therapy of these various conditions. The reader is referred to appropriate sections of standard pediatric textbooks for details.

Diagnostic etiologic considerations will include the historical points previously mentioned plus the addition of physical examination data which will implicate a specific causative agent. For example, in the child with moderate inspiratory stridor who does not have a history or physical signs compatible with epiglottitis or inhaled foreign body, the clinician will seek details as to the progression of the upper respiratory tract infection, the presence of similar inflammatory disease in other members of the child's family and classmates, and specific respiratory findings in the child, including the presence of upper respiratory inflammatory changes, otitis media, skin rash, and other manifestations suggestive of viral etiology. In each instance the clinician will have established hypotheses for which specific questions can be asked, the answers to which may indicate a specific etiologic agent.

In addition to etiologic considerations the clinician will refine his homeostatic analysis by such techniques as chest X-ray, blood gas determination, electrolyte determination and other measures of homeostatic balance.

At the conclusion of this diagnostic phase the clinician will have answered the primary question of the degree to which the process is life-threatening, will have established a reasonable homeostatic analysis, and will have begun specific etiologic diagnosis.

FURTHER ANALYSIS OF THE CHILD WITH EXPIRATORY WHEEZING

As previously mentioned, age is an important determinant in attempting to differentiate between bronchiolitis and allergic asthma. Clinical assessment of such infants will include historical information designed to reveal whether the current disease is part of a repetitive pattern or if it is an individual unique instance in this child's life. Epidemiologic evidence will be sought for similar disease in other members of the child's family and community, and a search will be instituted to reveal any environmental factors that may have played a role in the acute episode.

If the diagnosis suspected is asthma, environmental considerations become of paramount importance. Exact descriptions of the child's home environment, the exact circumstances under which the episode occurred, the prevailing environmental conditions in the air in the community, and other such factors will be delineated. If the child is sufficiently ill to require hospitalization, removal from such factors will be self-evident. The clinician will have time then to explore these relationships in greater detail and may even request or perform an evaluation of the environment on site.

Initially, however, the considerations are primarily homeostatic and etiologic. The degree to which the expiratory obstruction is impairing pulmonary function must be assessed. This is best done by a blood gas determination in the acute phase and, in some instances, by tests of pulmonary function. Since many children who have episodes of expiratory wheezing decrease their oral intake of fluids and electrolytes, estimation of dehydration and electrolyte imbalance are also sought. Infection plays a primary role in bronchiolitis and may be an incipient feature in asthma. As a result, historical, physical examination, and laboratory evidence for specific etiologic agents will be determined.

As indicated in the section on etiology above, there are many other potential causes of an acute wheezing episode. The diagnostician will search the history for clues that might indicate that cystic fibrosis or some of the other diseases are possible. Family history, previous medical history, response to therapy, associated symptoms and findings, and many other variables will be examined in an effort to identify clues to the presence of a more chronic or more basic disease that may account for the wheezing episode. If any of these hypotheses survive the initial elimination, specific laboratory tests for their presence are available and will be utilized. Again, it is beyond the scope of this chapter to delve into details of each of the diseases, and the reader is referred to the usual sources.

SUMMARY

In approaching the child with noisy respirations, the clinician must first distinguish between stridor and expiratory wheezing. Having established an approximate anatomic site for the production of the noisy respirations, the clinician then proceeds to make a judgement as to how urgent the necessity for intervention is, based on the degree to which life is threatened. Excessive obstruction at either end of the respiratory tract may require immediate measures to relieve the obstruction, guaranteeing sustenance of life and allowing a more leisurely pursuit of etiology and further definition of homeostatic imbalance. Subsequent analyses will delineate the degree to which the individual deviates from normal pulmonary function, and may result in identification of a specific etiologic cause or causes, which can then be corrected, modified or avoided in the future.

Chapter 15

The Child with a Seizure

INTRODUCTION

The occurrence of a convulsion in a child engenders considerable anxiety on the part of parents. The folklore surrounding convulsive disorders is ages old and has led to many misconceptions by parents and physicians alike.

A convulsive disorder is characterized by single or recurring episodes of convulsive movements or disturbances in feeling or behavior associated with the loss of consciousness. Although the final common pathway for the production of a convulsive disorder is excessive and uncontrolled electrical discharges from some portion of the brain, there are many different inciting factors that lead to such discharges. A convulsion is not a single entity that can be discussed in the absence of considerations of metabolic, fluid electrolyte, infectious, malignant and other considerations. However, at the other end of the spectrum it is clear that the acute management of convulsion does have common characteristics irrespective of the etiology. This latter fact has given rise to a false assumption in some diagnosticians' minds that convulsions in different children are similar in etiologic characteristics.

This chapter will attempt to delineate the etiologic differences in reference to the differential approach that diagnosticians must take. It will also emphasize the common characteristics of management of acute convul-sions and the reasoning underlying such management.

THE ETIOLOGY, EPIDEMIOLOGY AND CHARACTERISTICS OF CONVULSIVE DISORDERS

Types of Convulsions

Grand mal seizures involve generalized tonic and/or clonic movements of muscle groups associated with loss of consciousness. Concomitant with loss of consciousness the child will have strong muscular contractions principally involving the jaw muscles, the thoracic and abdominal musculature and the extremities. In some children a vague premonition (aura) may precede the convulsive episode. Commonly, urinary and fecal incontinence occur concomitant with seizure. The episode is extremely variable in length: some seizures last for less than a minute, and others last for hours. Loss of consciousness is universal, and recovery occurs shortly after the seizure ceases. The recovery may be complete with total amnesia for the episode or may be partial with residual drowsiness or even stupor. On occasion, dependent on the cause for the convulsion, coma may supervene.

Focal seizures often have the same characteristics as grand mal seizures except for their limitation to one part of the body. Commonly, one half of the body or one limb is involved, and occasionally, Jacksonian progression may be observed; i.e., the convulsion may begin with focal twitching of the distal portion of an extremity and spred proximally. It may end with involvement of that limb or may proceed to a more generalized convulsion. Focal seizures may be sensory in nature, involving paresthesias or numbness in the part, or may even be related to the special senses; e.g., repetitive visual sensations may occur.

Psychomotor seizures involve random or inappropriately purposeful movements during brief periods of altered consciousness. Many movements and activities are observed which may be simple or complex in nature. Some children will simply lapse into a "brown study," and others will have repetitive movements or behavior totally uncontrollable and unrelated to any purposeful activity. Most often brief, the psychomotor seizure may last up to several hours. Psychomotor seizures are believed to be due to abnormal discharges from the temporal lobe. One area in the temporal lobe, the infratemporal region, may result in an olfactory seizure in which the main characteristic is the perception of a peculiar odor. Other sensory manifestations may be observed, such as hearing a peculiar sound, tasting a peculiar taste, or various visual phenomena.

Petit mal or absence seizures are common in early childhood. There is a sudden loss of consciousness with staring, and, occasionally, rapid blinking of the eyelids may be observed. These seizures tend to be very brief, with consciousness regained immediately and a return to the fully normal state. In fact, the child may resume an activity, such as a conversation, that was interrupted by the attack. Petit mal seizures may be seen alone repetitively in a given child or may occur in combination with grand mal seizures.

Myoclonic seizures involve sudden momentary jerking movements of face, trunk or extremities. They may be single or repetitive in frequency and tend to occur just prior to going to sleep. There is no loss of consciousness, and they may occur with other forms of seizure activity.

In falling or akinetic seizures, there are sudden episodes of unconsciousness in which the child collapses. On occasion, the loss of muscle tone is limited to loss of head control alone. The episodes are brief, and full consciousness is immediately restored.

A particular form of myoclonic seizures, infantile spasms, consists of sudden jerking motions which involve flexion of the head and simultaneous flexion of the arms and legs. The myoclonic seizure is generalized, often occurring in series and separated by relaxation. Occasionally, other neurologic signs, such as nystagmus, and nonneurologic signs, such as cyanosis, may accompany the massive myoclonic jerk. Infantile spasms represent a specific clinical syndrome associated with many different antecedents. Central nervous system anomalies, cerebral maldevelopment, infection, immunization reactions, and a variety of metabolic disorders and other conditions may be associated with infantile spasms.

Rarely, other unusual forms of seizure-like activity may be observed. Recurrent abdominal pain, recurrent headache, tonic postural changes, and others are occasionally seen in individual children but will not be further considered in this chapter.

Age Relatedness

Grand mal seizures may be seen in any age from the newborn period through all stages of childhood and adolescence. Petit mal classically occurs in young children, often between the ages of 4 and 10 years. Psychomotor seizures tend to occur to slightly older children, particularly in the first few years of school. Infantile spasms are characteristically a problem observed in the first year of life and may be observed as late as 2 years of age. It is uncommon for infantile spasms to persist beyond 3 or 4 years of age. Focal and myoclonic seizure patterns may be observed at any age. Akinetic seizures most commonly are observed in the child who already walks and stands. If they occur in younger children, they may be difficult to detect and may be mistaken for other forms of seizure activity or for other conditions.

The Etiology of Seizures

A wide variety of causes of seizures are known. In this section we will attempt to delineate the major etiologic categories for convulsive disorders, recognizing that more than one mechanism may be responsible in an individual child.

Malformations of the cerebral cortex and other brain structures may develop in the course of fetal development. If the defect involves or inpinges upon areas of the cortex involved with motor or sensory activity, seizures may be observed during postnatal life. The seizures may result by direct effect of the particular lesion on an area of the cerebral cortex or may predispose that area to other stimuli, such as fever or drug effect, the seizures resulting from the other phenomena that occur to the child.

During delivery the infant may suffer anoxic insult with temporary or permanent injury to the cerebral cortex, and seizures may result.

Certain degenerative disorders of the central nervous system of unknown etiology may result in seizures. In contrast, some degenerative disorders are associated with biochemical abnormalities in protein, carbohydrate or lipid metabolism. These disorders may result in seizures because of direct effect of disease on neuronal integrity or because of secondary effects on metabolism. For example, some storage diseases may involve the neurons, leading to dysfunction and electrical discharge resulting in convulsions. On the other hand, if carbohydrate metabolic disorders are associated with hypoglycemia, one consequence may be hypoglycemic seizures in the infant.

Infections are a common cause of generalized seizures at any age but are particularly predominant in infancy. Fever accompanying a variety of infections may produce grand mal seizures in some susceptible children, irrespective of the underlying infection. On the other hand, specific infections involving the cerebral cortex, such as bacterial meningitis or encephalitis, may in themselves result in convulsions, irrespective of fever. In addition to acquired infections involving the brain and associated structures, congenital infection with a variety of viruses and parasites may result in a chronic syndrome with seizures as one manifestation.

The cerebral cortex is particularly suscep-

tible to alterations in fluid and electrolyte metabolism. Seizures can result from cerebral edema and generalized increased intracranial pressure, from specific swelling of neuronal cells secondary to water intoxication, from alterations in the flow and concentration of electrolytes without and within the neuronal cell, and from changes in the tonicity of blood passing through the brain. In addition, specific defects in serum concentrations of calcium, magnesium, glucose and other constituents may result in cerebral irritability, electrical discharge, and seizures. A specific metabolic deficiency, that of vitamin B_6 or pyridoxine, may develop in young infants, and its principle manifestation is grand mal seizures. This disorder can occur within a few days of life and throughout most of the first year.

Hepatic and renal disease may result in metabolic alterations which result in excessive cerebral irritability. In some renal diseases, hypertension may be a critical event, and hypertensive seizures may be observed.

A variety of poisons and drugs may act directly on the cerebral cortex in irritative fashion. Lead, thallium, organic phosphates, salicylates, steroids, a variety of phenothiazines, and other agents may evoke seizures in some children.

Hypertension from whatever cause may result in hypertensive encephalopathy in which seizures are a major manifestation. In childhood, acute glomerulonephritis or collagen vascular disease are the most common precursors of acute hypertension leading to convulsions.

Sufficient trauma at any age may lead to cerebral injury and irritability. Hemorrhage, contusion, laceration, interference with blood supply, and direct injury may occur during the birth process and result in seizures. In infancy, external injury, often the result of child abuse, may result in a variety of cerebral insults ranging from direct injury to the production of subdural hematomas and other forms of hemorrhage, and seizures can result. Older children may injure themselves accidentally with sufficient force to produce acute seizures or a chronic residual convulsive disorder.

Intracranial mass lesions ranging from benign tumors and subdural collections to malignancies and brain abcesses can result in seizure activity, depending on the localization. *It is uncommon in young children and infants for seizures to be a primary or first manifestation of intracerebral masses.* This is in contradistinction to adult life in which seizures may herald the presence of a brain tumor.

A variety of vascular disorders of either congenital or acquired origin may cause cerebral irritability and convulsions. Such lesions as arteriovenous aneurysms, cerebral arterial thrombosis, or embolization are examples of this form of convulsive etiology.

Finally, some children will have seizures due to unknown causes. In fact, the bulk of recurrent afebrile convulsive disorders in infants and children have no discernible etiology and have come to be known collectively as *idiopathic epilepsy.* In some series, more than half of the children who display convulsions of any type fall into this category. As we shall see, the distinction between this group and those with specific etiologic designation is the major reason for a systematic approach to diagnosis and for a diligent search for clues which may establish a specific cause as opposed to assigning the child to the idiopathic group.

Of interest, as newer research methods develop, a portion of the idiopathic group becomes assigned to a specific etiologic category. For example, prior to the appreciation of B_6 metabolism and its necessity for cerebral cortical integrity, children with this disorder were assigned to the idiopathic epileptic group. In some children physical phenomena in their environment appear to be causally related to individual seizures. This group is still classified as idiopathic despite the fact that the particular sensory stimulation is known.

Other Considerations in Seizure Disorders

It is clear that not all individuals are predisposed to convulsions as an expression of cerebral irritability under a variety of stimuli. Extensive investigation of genetic patterns has been made in an attempt to delineate the susceptible individual from the nonsusceptible. Of most reliability is the family history of convulsive disorders in siblings, parents or bloodline relatives. It has been estimated that more than one third of children with idiopathic epilepsy and approximately one half of children with febrile seizures have such a family history. Genetic studies have suggested autosomal dominance with incomplete penetrance as the probable underlying mechanism for such susceptibility. However, even cursory examination of the list of etiologies above will indicate that to overemphasize genetic susceptibility would be simplistic at best.

Despite the association of specific electroencephalographic patterns with the various types of epilepsy, electroencephalography itself has not assisted in delineating the various etiologic causes except in a very few instances.

The diagnostician is basically left with the dilemma of providing immediate care for the child who has a seizure disorder and then attempting a systematic sorting out of the various causes before he assigns the patient to the idiopathic epilepsy group. In a discussion such as this one, it is all too easy to consider convulsions as a single entity to be dealt with in an organized fashion. In reality, an individual child presenting with a convulsion may direct the physician by virtue of specific clues to any of the categories above without the need for an exhaustive differential diagnosis. This point will be made repeatedly inasmuch as it is critical to understanding the diagnostic process.

THE DIAGNOSTIC PROCESS IN CONVULSIVE DISORDERS IN INFANCY AND CHILDHOOD

Although the first test confronting the physician who is dealing with a convulsive disorder is management of the acute episode, we will reverse the process here and consider etiologic differentiation first. Of critical importance in the initial approach to a child with single or repetitive seizures is accurate description of the seizure and categorization insofar as it is possible. The reasons for such distinction are related to the frequency of certain types of seizures in certain etiologic categories. For example, the young infant with recurrent seizures of a focal nature has a more likely probability of having a metabolic or developmental cause than some of the other etiologic categories.

Thus, the first test that the physician faces is a complete and accurate description of the seizure. This is often made difficult because this seizure activity may be very brief and most often is not observed by the clinician. He is relying almost totally on a description by the parents or caretakers of the seizure activity. In one recent instance in my own experience, I encountered a child who had had multiple diagnostic examinations and multiple attempts at etiologic assessment in whom no single seizure had ever been observed by any of the physicians who were attempting to reach diagnostic conclusions. The striking factor in this instance was that the period during which the seizures had occurred was 3½ years. In every instance the seizure was manifest only at home or at school and never in a medical examiner's presence. This phenomenon is more common than is appreciated and is one of the rare instances in medicine in which the disease for which an explanation is sought has no observable manifestations to the diagnostician. In this child's case, multiple examinations indicated normalcy. This anecdote does not mean that the child did not have seizures. Nor does it mean that the diagnostician must be paralyzed unless personal observation of seizure activity occurs. It does mean that an extremely careful history must be taken in most instances and that detailed documentation of a nonskilled person's observations be made. Each of the seizure types are sufficiently characteristic that careful documentation is possible by history. If one considers the extent of diagnostic techniques available to the diagnostician, the necessity for careful historical documentation should be obvious.

Factors in the history, apart from description of individual seizure activity, include the age of the child at the onset of the seizures, the frequency of episodes, the duration of episodes, careful environmental history to reveal any possible exposures to inciting factors such as poisons or drugs, careful delineation of the stages of development including prenatal influences, and a careful family history for both seizures and other manifestations of disease which might have an inherited or familial basis. In addition, it is important to delineate prior therapy, particularly if the seizures have been repetitive. It is important also to ascertain any home remedies that might have been employed, as certain subcultures will utilize a variety of herbal and dietary prescriptions that abound in folklore.

In acute seizures in which fever is a component, history must also focus on the particular infection that produced the fever. A common dilemma for the diagnostician is that of the proper approach to the child with febrile seizure. The dilemma is created by the knowledge, on one hand, that fever alone can produce seizures without any direct infectious involvement of the central nervous system. On the other hand, the fever and convulsion may be symptomatic of early bacterial or viral meningitis. Obviously, if bacterial meningitis is present, it is urgent that it be diagnosed and treated. Since febrile convulsions occur most commonly in children between 6 months and 4 years of age and affect a sizable portion of our childhood population, it is clear that the dilemma takes on significant proportions. The earlier part of this age spectrum is also the period during which bacterial meningitis occurs, thus heightening the urgency for accurate and specific diagnosis.

Obviously, historical features which would be compatible with meningitis will be sought, such as the degree of irritability and playfulness of the child and symptoms associated with increased intracranial pressure, such as vomiting. As will be apparent in further discussion, the physical examination also becomes critical. However, it is pertinent to mention that a large majority of these children will have a negative physical examination and a history compatible only with a respiratory infection that produced the fever. It is precisely in this group of children that the diagnostic dilemma is joined. We will consider this problem further at a later point in the discussion.

The physical examination in the child who has had a seizure consists of two parts. On the one hand, the clinician will do a more thorough neurologic examination than in children without neurologic symptoms. What is being sought are signs of increased intracranial pressure, focal neurologic deficits, and gross abnormalities in motor, sensory and equilibrium functions. Complicating this assessment is the frequent occurrence of so-called Todd's paralysis. It is not uncommon for children who have had grand mal or focal seizures to be left with a residual weakness, often of a single extremity or involving one half of the body. This is a temporary phenomenon that does not have diagnostic significance in terms of a focal lesion in the cerebral cortex. All children who exhibit this form of postictal paralysis raise in the diagnostician's mind the possibility that a focal lesion is indeed present. Only continued observation and, in some instances, further diagnostic procedures will assist in this determination.

The other half of the physical examination will involve careful search for clues as to underlying disease. In acute single convulsions attention will be focused on concomitant infections, on hypertension and renal disease, and on evidence of trauma or other acute insults. With repetitive seizures the examination will also extend to a search for clues of underlying metabolic or other disorders.

One form of acute febrile seizure that is often confusing to the pediatrician is the occurrence of a single grand mal seizure in a mildly febrile patient who appears quite ill. There may have been a previous complaint of abdominal pain or vomiting, but often no specific gastrointestinal symptom is present. During the course of the evaluation of the seizure the child often will have bloody stool and thus announce the presence of bacillary dysentery secondary to shigellosis. *Shigella* has a specific exotoxin which produces convulsions in some children, which convulsions may occur prior to the onset of diarrhea.

In many children, completion of the data collection by history and physical examination will be sufficient to establish hypotheses as to cause of seizures. It may be clearly established that the infant has a high probability of bacterial meningitis or sufficient head trauma to suggest intracranial bleeding or some other specific diagnostic delineation. In such instances the clinician is guided towards further diagnostic procedures by the specificity of his hypotheses.

Obviously, if bacterial meningitis is suspected, the next order of diagnostic business is to examine the cerebrospinal fluid. In such instances the sequence of diagnostic testing becomes of critical concern. As has been discussed earlier in this volume, such sequencing can be of critical nature to the child. In the instance of a child who has had a febrile seizure in which excessive irritability has been detected both by history and by observation, but in whom no specific signs of increased intracranial pressure or meningeal irritation are evident, the clinician may be tempted to employ nonspecific screening tests. Often the rationale for such proceeding is the uncertainty of the presence of bacterial meningitis and the desire to increase the clinician's judgement as to whether lumbar puncture should be attempted. This is an example of potentially faulty reasoning, since the answer to the question, "Is bacterial meningitis present or not?" can only adequately be answered by examination of the spinal fluid. Therefore, the correct sequence is to sample the cerebrospinal fluid first. In actual practice many clinicians prefer to obtain such tests as a chest X-ray or total white blood cell count and differential to rule out pneumonia or to indicate the presence of a bacterial infection. It is my view that this is unnecessary delay in answering the basic question, which is, "Is this child's seizure due to bacterial meningitis?" As was mentioned earlier, many children with febrile seizures will pose this dilemma to the clinician.

Obviously, any generalization will be weakened in the specific instance, and it is didactically dangerous to advocate a single course of action. In fact, a lively debate has occurred among experienced clinicians and other experts in this area as to the necessity for utilizing lumbar puncture in such individuals. There is no clear resolution, although many of us, including the author, lean towards examination of the spinal fluid with the first febrile seizure episode and with any subsequent ones that have the least suspicion that cerebral irritability or increased intracranial pressure is present. Our reasoning is that the lumbar puncture is a relatively innocuous procedure when compared in risk/management fashion to the hazard of not diagnosing bacterial meningitis. Those of us advocating this course of action must recognize that a large number of normal children (in relation to children with bacterial meningitis) will be subjected to lumbar puncture to garner the few who have early meningitis. We feel this risk is worth taking.

In many instances of a single seizure the child is not febrile and does not have signs of infection in the respiratory or other systems. The usual clinical scenario includes a relatively normal-appearing child who may be slightly drowsy having been brought to the physician's attention after the afebrile seizure has ended. The history and physical examination in such children is almost always normal (except with the occasional presence of postictal paralysis). In such children, little need be done on the first encounter, and subsequent diagnostic tests can be accomplished in more leisurely fashion. Armed with the knowledge that many afebrile seizures are of metabolic, fluid and electrolyte, or renal origin, many routine approaches have been developed towards diagnostic screening.

It is not uncommon for some diagnosticians to proclaim that every child who has had an afebrile seizure should have as a minimum a total white blood cell count and differential, serum electrolyte determination, calcium, magnesium and phosphate levels in the serum, a blood glucose determination, and a renal battery to include at least blood urea nitrogen and examination of the urinary sediment. In addition, some clinicians would add radiographs of the skull and long bones and an examination of cerebrospinal fluid. Such routines are based on the assumption that the hypotheses generated by a single afebrile seizure are those of the multiple etiologic categories considered earlier. They argue that these disorders are undetectable in many instances by historical or physical examination data and must be routinely addressed by specific laboratory testing.

Large-scale studies of such approaches again illustrate their futility, since most children have normal values for these determinations. From the risk/management standpoint it is difficult to argue against a small battery of screening tests of low yield being employed in every such child. For the child with the rare metabolic cause, for example, detection is of invaluable assistance. Unfortunately, overinterpretation of minor laboratory abnormalities unrelated to seizure production also occurs. For example, the diagnosis of hypoglycemia may be made on a marginally low, but normal, glucose determination, and because of the seriousness with which seizures are regarded, major alterations made in a child's diet with the false assumption that hypoglycemia is present. Of course, one may argue that this is simply error of interpretation and not of commission, in that the test itself was proper to obtain but that a correct interpretation should have been placed on the laboratory value.

My own view is that a minimum of laboratory testing of this type should be employed for most children with a single afebrile seizure without any clinical clues pointing in any specific direction. If the child has another seizure or if in continued observation additional historical or physical examination data accumulate, application of specific diagnostic tests is warranted.

The most frequently disputed diagnostic approach concerns the necessity for obtaining roentgenograms of the skull and electroencephalograms in children with afebrile seizures. Virtually every one agrees that an electroencephalogram should be performed, particularly since distinctive patterns may be associated with certain types of seizures. Unfortunately, in acute episodes, disordered electrical activity may persist for some days following an acute seizure irrespective of its etiology. Thus, the electroencephalogram, if obtained, should be performed at some interval from the acute seizure; usually an interval of 1 to 6 weeks is advocated.

On the other hand, some neurologists argue that a normal electroencephalogram immediately postseizure is a strong argument against idiopathic epilepsy or specific focal lesions. The frailty in this argument is that since most electroencephalograms will be nonspecifically disordered, a repeat examination will be necessary, and thus, both inconvenience and expense to the patient have been incurred. My own view is that in most instances an electroencephalogram should be delayed unless there are compelling clues which suggest that it must be done. For example, in a temporal lobe seizure with persistent symptomatology one may wish to identify an abnormal focus that may be related to a specific infection, such as herpes simplex encephalitis, or to a mass lesion in the region.

Skull roentgenograms are of little diagnostic value in most children with seizure disorders. It is the rare child who will demonstrate intracranial calcifications or other evidence of significant intracranial disease. This procedure is of sufficiently low yield that it is my belief, and that of many neurologists, that it should not be performed routinely in these circumstances.

The recent addition to our armamentarium of computerized axial tomography (CAT scans) has further complicated the diagnostic approach. Many clinicians mindlessly obtain this expensive and elaborate procedure in every child who has a seizure disorder. They take such action despite the fact that convulsions seldom herald an intracranial lesion in childhood. CAT scans in these circumstances are best at detecting mass lesions for which the probability is extremely low. It is my best estimate that the newness and uniqueness of this procedure has engendered the excessive use in children with afebrile convulsions and that continued experience and practice will relegate it to a more appropriate position. CAT scans should be obtained in children in whom there is sufficient evidence to warrant an hypothesis of space-occupying lesion or other diagnosis that may be detected by CAT scan. It is unwarranted to employ this technique routinely in every child who has had an afebrile seizure.

Obviously, selected specific diagnostic procedures will be and should be entertained in circumstances strongly suggestive of underlying specific conditions. For example, if a seizure is accompanied by specific and persistent focal findings, the use of CAT scanning and subsequent arteriography or other diagnostic procedures may well be indicated. In an infant with focal seizures and evidence of delayed development or growth, one may wish to employ elaborate metabolic screening tests, such as search for organic acidemias and for aminoacidopathies. In a child with a seizure and evidence of increased intracranial pressure in whom a history of pica is obtained, one may wish to screen for lead levels as well as to examine long bones for so-called lead lines.

THE MANAGEMENT OF THE INITIAL SEIZURE

In contradistinction to etiologic thinking, the management of an acute seizure still in progress at the time the child is brought to the physician's attention involves predominantly homeostatic reasoning. The convulsion can lead to anoxia, and an aspiration of gastric contents may occur. In addition, the child may injure himself by various involuntary movements. The tongue may be bitten and severe bleeding result, or the child may fall from an examining table during the episode. As a result, initial attention must be directed towards maintenance of an adequate airway and oxygenation, appropriate restraint of the child during the seizure, and some method to insure that damage is not done to oral structures.

Most seizures will terminate spontaneously and in a reasonably short period of time, and no specific therapy need be entertained. In others the seizure may be prolonged, and fear of cerebral anoxia paramount. Such children should have appropriate anticonvulsant medication. It is beyond the scope of this chapter to discuss the selection of individual medications. The purpose in employment of such therapy is to terminate the seizure without undue side effects. Judgement as to the necessity for this is conditioned by the seizure itself, by the degree to which cerebral anoxia is a potential problem and, to some extent, by the underlying condition. For example, if the child has bacterial meningitis, the seizures may be prolonged and severe and may result from cerebral irritation directly or from increased intracranial pressure or cerebral edema. In such instances it may be desirable to reduce cerebral edema by an appropriate osmotic agent simultaneously with an attempt to terminate the seizures with appropriate anticonvulsant medication. In addition, it is essential to initiate therapy for the meningitis to reverse the irritative process by bringing the infection under control. In status epilepticus, irrespective of cause, it is necessary to terminate the seizures in order to prevent harm to the patient. This condition is one of the few true medical emergencies and must be recognized, and all of the above measures employed to insure oxygenation, avoid injury and terminate the seizure.

If fever is a major component for the seizure and if the symptoms persist, measures to control fever may be necessary. It is important to remember that even with prolonged febrile episodes the seizure activity may only occur with the first elevation in body temperature and not persist. Therefore, it is important not to be overly aggressive in one's approach, causing more damage by the measures designed to control the potential for seizure than the potential merits.

If a seizure occurs in association with a known metabolic state, such as diabetes with insulin therapy, it may be wise to administer intravenous glucose even prior to adequate testing of this hypothesis. Prolonged hypoglycemic seizures can be destructive, and the reasoning underlying this approach is that intravenous glucose is harmless and may be essential in the therapy of hypoglycemia.

In certain toxic seizures in which increased intracranial pressure is a major component, cautious but definite reduction in intracranial pressure may be essential. Concomitantly, if the toxin has been introduced orally, one may out of necessity make efforts to reduce further absorption and to rid the body of unabsorbed toxins present in the gastrointestinal tract.

If one suspects an intracranial mass lesion, immediate neurosurgical intervention may be indicated.

It can be seen from this discussion that critical determinates of acute initial management include a rapid and thorough assessment of the potential for damage that the convulsive episode displays. In addition, some etiologic reasoning must be employed, although the effect is a return to normal homeostasis. The clinician is initially interested in returning the child to a safer homeostatic level and only secondarily interested in the specific etiologic cause. In some instances, obviously, the two blend imperceptively, as is the case, for example, in bacterial meningitis with increased intracranial pressure secondary to cerebral edema. In such an instance the clinician manages abnormal homeostasis at the same time that he initiates specific therapy following an appropriate and specific diagnostic pathway.

Chapter 16

The Child with Abdominal Pain

INTRODUCTION

Acute abdominal pain is one of the most common symptoms encountered in pediatric practice. Chronic recurring abdominal pain, although less frequent, is a common complaint in school-age and adolescent individuals.

Abdominal pain arises from perception of stimuli within the abdominal cavity, from the surrounding abdominal musculature and from causes distant from the abdomen. Several mechanisms are responsible for the perception of pain. Smooth muscle spasm due to stretching or irritation of the gastrointestinal tract may result in visceral signals being sent to the corresponding segment in the spinal cord. The pain is then perceived by the same sensory components and is usually referred to an appropriate site on the abdominal wall. Similar mechanisms apply to spasm and irritation in the genitourinary and biliary tracts.

This type of pain tends to be diffuse and nondescript without immediate localization. Often the child will indicate a general region of the abdomen and be unable to pinpoint the pain. The pain can be acute and cramp-like or can be more constant and dull. Pain can also arise from irritation of the peritoneal surfaces. The serosa is liberally supplied with sensitive nerve endings, and inflammatory changes result in irritation with the percep-

tion of a dull, often severe and generalized, pain. Further, stretching of the capsule of the liver may result in pain localized to that organ. This is often dull, aching and severe with a persistent quality that is exaggerated by pressure over the liver.

Pain arising within the gastrointestinal tract may be referred to specific sites in the abdomen. The upper third of the gastrointestinal tract, including the stomach, duodenum and a portion of the jejunum will refer pain to the epigastrium. Jejunal and ileal pain and pain arising in and around the cecum will often be referred to the umbilicus or midabdomen, and pain in the distal third of the gastrointestinal tract will often be referred to the suprapubic area. Localized organ pain tends to be referred to specific areas of the abdomen. Liver pain is predominantly in the right upper quadrant, as is the pain of biliary disease. Pain of renal origin may frequently be referred to the flank and down into the inguinal area. Painful pelvic organs will generally have pain referred to the lower abdomen or the perineum.

Despite the neat localizations, it is often true in children that many different causes of abdominal pain in many different sites are referred directly to the area surrounding the umbilicus. It is a frustrating experience for diagnosticians to be unable to get a child to localize pain other than pointing directly to the belly-button. This may result because most acute abdominal pain and causes of chronic pain in children involve those areas of the bowel with referral patterns to the midabdomen. It may also be because young children are less concerned with the specifics of their pain and more concerned with the discomfort it produces. Thus, the vague referral to the midabdomen may be more apparent than real. Whichever mechanism is predominant, the fact remains that for many disorders in young children, no specific localization other than the midabdomen will be volunteered.

Some diagnosticians will make a great deal of the character of the abdominal pain in relation to the precipitating cause. Most of this experience has been gleaned from adolescents and adults and in diseases such as renal colic and biliary tract disease which are relatively uncommon in childhood. As a result, the characteristic pattern of pain described in textbooks may not fit an individual situation with a young child. This has proved particularly frustrating in the diagnosis of acute appendicitis in which all types of pain localized to the midabdomen can be described.

The task facing the clinician in the diagnosis of acute and chronic abdominal pain is to sort out potentially devastating and progressive illnesses from those which have a more leisurely pace and will not eventuate into serious or life-threatening consequences. One of the true frustrations in pediatric practice is the occurrence of acute appendicitis in children under the age of 2. The frustration is occasioned by the lack of specificity of the syndrome with the result that many such children present only after rupture of the appendix and ensuing peritonitis. It is just such events that frustrate the clinician as he attempts to sort out correctable causes, such as acute appendicitis, from the myriad of forerunners of abdominal pain of different significance.

THE CAUSE OF ACUTE ABDOMINAL PAIN

In any consideration of acute abdominal pain, age differentiation must be taken into account. The infant has a completely different variety of causes from that in the older child and adolescent. In essence, functional physiologic causes of abdominal pain and structural causes due to a variety of mechanical conditions predominate in the etiology of acute abdominal pain.

The most frequent cause of abdominal pain in the young infant is termed colic. It has its onset in the first few weeks of life and usually does not occur after 5 or 6 months of age. The infant manifests behavior indicative of irritability and seemingly localized to the abdomen by the commonly observed thrusting of legs onto the abdominal surface. In many infants it's a daily occurrence, frequently lasting for several hours, often at or around suppertime. The infant may cry, fret, or manifest constant motor activity during the episode, and although a variety of maneuvers will be attempted, few are successful in reversing the irritability. During the episode the infant frequently will flex the legs onto the abdomen, which has led most observers to believe that intestinal spasm is responsible for colic. This would appear to be a physiologic disorder somehow related to the infant's temperament and the family constellation. It does not occur in all infants and is of variable severity and duration among those infants in which it does occur.

A large variety of structural and obstructive disorders in the gastrointestinal tract will produce acute episodes of abdominal pain. These include volvulus, intussusception and incarcerated hernias, both internal and external. In addition, intestinal obstruction secondary to congenital bands or membranes or due to pyloric stenosis may manifest as both abdominal pain and vomiting.

Acute appendicitis does occur in infancy and will manifest itself in similar fashion to colic. That is, the infant may display increased irritability and some thrusting of the legs onto the abdomen and may have fever and either diarrhea or constipation with or without vomiting. This disease is extremely difficult to differentiate from other causes of abdominal pain. Indeed, appendicitis may not even be suspected if irritability is the major or sole manifestation of the inflammatory process.

Many infants exhibit features compatible

with abdominal pain at a time when infections are present elsewhere in the body. It is not uncommon for infants and young children to complain of abdominal pain during a bout of acute upper respiratory tract infection.

Abdominal pain may also be secondary to the ingestion of toxic substances or to inflammation of the gastrointestinal tract secondary to gastroenteritis. Least commonly, peritonitis may occur in young infants secondary to perforation of a viscus and result in severe abdominal pain.

In older children, infection and inflammatory diseases are the predominant reasons for acute abdominal pain. Gastroenteritis is the most frequent cause and may be viral, bacterial or toxic in origin.

In many infections of the upper respiratory tract, abdominal pain is an acute and persistent feature. In the past, it was believed that so-called mesenteric adenitis was responsible for such abdominal pain. This concept evolved from the observation that children operated upon for acute appendicitis were discovered to have a normal appendix but greatly enlarged and swollen mesenteric lymph nodes. It is uncertain if the mesenteric adenitis is actually responsible for the abdominal pain in such individuals.

Acute appendicitis, of course, will produce abdominal pain secondary to inflammation and obstruction and even rupture of the appendix. Another common cause of abdominal pain are inflammation localized to one part of the gastrointestinal tract that may be abnormal. For example, a Meckel's diverticulum may ulcerate and become inflamed and produce abdominal pain. In inflammatory diseases such as regional enteritis and ulcerative collitis, abdominal pain is often a prominent feature and may present a difficult diagnostic dilemma at the onset of the disease.

Abdominal pain in older children can also result from involvement of other organs. Abdominal pain is frequent in acute glomerulonephritis and acute pyelonephritis. It also occurs in primary viral hepatitis and in the variety of diseases that may produce inflammation of the liver, such as mononucleosis. Although infrequent in childhood, gallbladder disease, either inflammatory or obstruc-

tive in nature, can occur, and severe right upper quadrant pain may be experienced. Inflammation in the genital tract is occasionally seen ranging from tubo-ovarian abscess to such mechanical causes as torsion of the spermatic cord.

A common cause of abdominal pain is acute bacterial pneumonia. In this instance the abdominal pain may be the result of direct lymphatic spread to the parietal peritoneum or may be related to bacterial toxins released into the blood which cause functional disability in the gastrointestinal tract.

A frequent cause of abdominal pain in school-age children is that which accompanies acute streptococcal respiratory infections. Vomiting may also occur, and on occasion, the diagnosis of acute appendicitis must be entertained despite the presence of clear-cut streptococcal exudative tonsillar pharyngitis. Mechanical causes of abdominal pain are not frequent in early childhood unless a preexisting lesion which has been silent for many years becomes involved in an inflammatory or other process. For example, a child may have asymptomatic duplication of the gastrointestinal tract, and only with acute gastroenteritis will obstructive changes become obvious.

In any child who has had previous abdominal surgery the possibility of intestinal obstruction at any interval after surgery must be considered. A variety of poisons may lead to abdominal pain, ranging from lead to a host of medications.

Rarely, abdominal pain may be the manifestation of a systemic disease, such as sickle cell anemia or diabetes mellitus. Even more rarely, porphyria may have to be considered.

At all ages, constipation may produce acute abdominal pain. However, this is often a wastebasket diagnosis which is utilized when other explanation can be found. A few children with acute constipation manifest all the signs and symptoms of an acute abdomen. Upon removal of the fecal contents, the symptoms disappear and do not recur unless there is a reason for constipation to recur.

Ulcer disease is a distinctly uncommon entity in pediatrics. However, in some areas of the country, exuberant radiologists and clinicians will diagnose peptic ulcer more frequently than appears warranted by careful study. Similarly, gallbladder disease is uncommon in childhood, and except in certain clinical states such as hemolytic anemia, gallstones do not develop during childhood, and obstructive biliary tract disease is rare. Similarly, renal colic secondary to stone production is uncommon except in certain metabolic disorders in which stone formation is one component of urinary excretion of an abnormal metabolite.

THE ETIOLOGY OF RECURRENT AND CHRONIC ABDOMINAL PAIN

Most often, chronic or recurrent abdominal pain is not diagnosable unless there have been at least three separate episodes spaced over a period of many months. The most common cause of recurrent abdominal pain in childhood is not related to structural, inflammatory or pathophysiologic dysfunction within the abdomen.

The most common syndrome encountered appears to be related to maladjustment and behavioral disorder in the child. In no way does this negate the impact on the child and the family or the significance of the disorder. It does complicate the approach to such a child, since only a very few will have correctable lesions that should be identified. The vast majority of such children will require diligent attention to their personality development and their environmental and interpersonal relationships. The abdominal pain in such individuals is often diffuse or may be localized to the umbilicus. The episodes are accompanied by considerable disability and may result in prolonged absences from school or other activities. Usually the only symptom is abdominal pain, although, on occasion, vomiting or constipation may occur.

Typically, the child is between 5 years of age and adolescence and is completely well between episodes. The pain tends to be crampy, rarely lasting more than a few hours. Most often the pain is unassociated with other factors in the environment, such as food intake, activity or defecation, but in some children a particular pattern develops that is repeated for that child. Headache, dizziness, anorexia and constipation occur occasionally, and the child is often described as being pale

and appearing sick during the episode. Rarely, intercurrent fever occurs concomitant with the abdominal pain. Growth is almost never impaired, nor is development. However, schooling may be adversely affected, and the child may be in academic difficulty as a result of frequent absences.

Other causes of recurrent abdominal pain include an enormous number of possibilities. It would be impossible in a text such as this to catalogue all of the causes of recurrent abdominal pain in children. Instead, we will try to enumerate the major categories and focus on a few entities that are sufficiently common to merit your consideration.

Gastrointestinal causes will include a variety of chronic infections, such as amebiasis and giardiasis. Noninfectious inflammatory causes include regional enteritis and ulcerative colitis. In regional enteritis the episodes of abdominal pain may have been preceded by undiagnosed periods of fever. Conversely, the onset may be heralded by fever, abdominal pain and diarrhea simultaneously. In ulcerative colitis the abdominal pain is often associated with the onset of mucoid bloody diarrhea, and tenesmus, pain on defecation, frequently accompanies the syndrome.

Mechanical causes may also be present and undiagnosed for years in children with recurrent abdominal pain. Conditions such as volvulus and internal hernia may produce intermittent episodes of colicky abdominal pain which disappear when the primary cause corrects itself temporarily. A Meckel's diverticulum with intermittent ulceration usually produces painless abdominal bleeding but, on occasion, will produce recurrent pain.

Chronic constipation syndromes, including both functional and structural abnormalities of the colon, may result in intermittent episodes of abdominal pain. In such instances the history will reveal the lack or infrequency of bowel movements and provide a valuable clue as to the underlying cause.

Chronic renal disease, especially inflammation in minor degrees of obstruction, may, on occasion, present with abdominal pain as a prominent or sole feature. More commonly, chronic pyelonephritis will be accompanied by acute episodes of urinary tract infection with characteristic symptomatology.

Chronic inflammatory changes in other intra-abdominal organs, such as the gallbladder or pancreas, are distinctly uncommon in childhood. Nonabdominal causes include all of the metabolic, hematologic and autoimmune diseases mentioned above in the discussion of acute pain. Thus, sickle cell disease, diabetes mellitus, epilepsy and collagen vascular disease may be manifest as recurrent episodes of abdominal pain.

A variety of cyclic diseases may involve fever and abdominal pain as prominent manifestations. In many instances our understanding of these diseases is incomplete or lacking. A few children will have familial patterns of cyclic episodes of abdominal pain in which all attempts at diagnosis fail.

It is of interest that as few as 5% of children beyond infancy who present with chronic or recurrent abdominal pain will have a specific, identifiable etiology. All of the others will fall into the category that appears to involve personality disorders or behavioral or environmental abnormalities.

THE DIAGNOSTIC APPROACH TO THE CHILD WITH ABDOMINAL PAIN

It should be clear from consideration of the multiple etiologies and the epidemiology of abdominal pain that in most instances of acute pain a specific cause is present which may be discernible. In contrast, in most instances of chronic or recurrent pain a specific cause will not be found. This generalization will serve as a guideline for us as we consider our approach to children with the two types of presentation.

In acute abdominal pain the basic search is for inflammatory or mechanical processes or a combination of these as cause for the abdominal pain. Data collection should focus on establishing, to the extent possible, the nature, localization and referral of the abdominal pain. Unfortunately, in many young children this will result in frustration, as the pain will be described as "all over" or will be localized to the periumbilical area. The diagnostician will also seek out data indicative of infection within the abdominal vault or at some distance from it.

Of particular importance in delineating mechanical causes is the search for evidence of obstruction and for the intermittent colicky nature of the pain. In some children intra-abdominal anomalies are associated with other congenital defects. Detection of cardiac, genital, limb or other defects may lead the clinician to suspect a gastrointestinal or genitourinary defect as well.

In most instances of acute abdominal pain the clinician has uppermost in his mind the necessity for ruling out or establishing the presence of appendicitis. The classic approach has been to use a combination of historical, physical examination and laboratory data to place the child at risk in a highly probable, possible, or improbable category.

In the highly probable category, children who exhibit typical progression from periumbilical pain to localization of pain in the right lower quadrant associated with anorexia, low-grade fever and no signs of gastroenteritis will be excellent candidates. If they, in addition, have mild elevation of their white blood cell count with some shift to the left and a negative urinalysis, they will be considered for operative intervention. Children of school age and adolescents often display a characteristic enough picture to be considered in this high-risk category.

In the improbable category at the other end of the spectrum are children who do not have classic historical findings and who may have associated fever or evidence of infection in the respiratory or gastrointestinal tract. If, in addition, their white blood cell count is not characteristic or if urinalysis reveals the possibility of urinary tract infection, the clinician will relegate them to the low-risk category.

Intermediate in position between these extremes are the children who display indeterminate features. Their abdominal pain may remain localized to the umbilicus or may be in a noncharacteristic pattern due to the location of the appendix. Thus, such children may complain of back pain or pelvic pain or may even have irritative symptoms referable to the urinary tract if the appendix abuts on the urinary bladder or ureters. They may have considerable vomiting and even some diarrhea. Their laboratory values may be consistent or inconsistent with the diagnosis.

In all such categories, physical examination may be a critical determinant. An experienced primary care physician or surgeon may have increased confidence in the category in which the child is placed, based on the presence or absence of certain physical findings. In the classic instance, depression of the abdomen in the right lower quadrant will result in severe tenderness. Localized muscle spasm with guarding and rebound may be present. Both abdominal and rectal examination may reveal the presence of an extremely tender localized area or even what appears to be a mass. If one then combines the characteristic historical features and a convincing physical examination, the decision to perform surgical exploration is straightforward.

In some children, however, irrespective of the history, the physical examination is nondescript. Abdominal pain is generalized and not localized to any site, there is absence or variability in muscular rigidity or rebound, and the rectal examination does not produce specific localized tenderness. These children may still have acute appendicitis, but a period of observation may be warranted before surgical intervention is considered. In these cases the clinician establishes an hypothesis of possible acute appendicitis and utilizes reevaluation with additional data collection as the primary test. In some instances the clinician may choose to use such techniques as roentgenologic examination to assist him during this period of observation. However, the findings may not be helpful, and observation may be much more critical. Of course, if a fecalith in the appendix or a localized-absence-of-gas pattern is present, the balance may be tipped towards surgical intervention.

Even in instances of assignment to the improbable category, continued observation is essential. A very few of these children will, in fact, have acute appendicitis despite the nondescript nature and even misleading signs and symptoms. Only by continuous reevaluation can individuals be sorted out from this group or become more classical or more suspect as time goes on.

The infant with acute appendicitis represents a very specific problem. Typically, the characteristic signs and symptoms are not present, and the child poses a diagnostic and therapeutic dilemma. On the one hand, it is obviously desirable to remove an inflamed appendix in a young child, since perforation is likely and disability and even mortality will increase with the passage of time. On the other hand, one does not wish to subject an ill child without appendicitis to a major anesthetic and surgical experience. Often the only course to follow is repeated and frequent examinations in a hospital in an attempt to detect any signs suggestive of acute appendicitis. The experienced clinician may wish to examine such an infant under anesthesia in order to obtain better data on which to make a judgement. Least desirable is to send the infant home if this tentative hypothesis has been made. It is far better that the infant be subjected to an unnecessary 12 to 24 hours of observation in a hospital setting than to have his appendix rupture at some distance from medical care. In every experienced clinician's practice, enough instances are encountered in which the diagnosis of appendicitis is missed in such infants that overcaution is warranted and a conservative approach should always be followed.

In children within whom recurrent episodes of abdominal pain are the predominant feature the clinician's approach should be quite different. In these instances, diagnostic intervention and therapeutic endeavors should only rarely be utilized. Armed with the knowledge that most instances of recurrent abdominal pain are related to personality, environmental or familial disorders, the physician's attention should be dedicated to establishing that hypothesis rather than to ruling out the uncommon and unlikely possibilities enumerated above.

There is a sound therapeutic reason for this, quite apart from the expense, inconvenience and discomfort of the patient who is spared. In a child in whom abdominal pain is an expression of psychosocial forces, the diagnostician may emphasize the symptoms by unnecessary and unwarranted procedures. It is an all-too-common occurrence that such children have elaborate gastrointestinal and blood studies in which a cycle is created of expectation on the part of the child and the family that a cause is present and will be found. This cycle, then, has repetitive episodes in which the diagnostician increases the tempo of his search. All of us have encountered instances in which a patient was actually submitted to exploratory laparotomy with virtually no indication and a host of negative diagnostic tests preceding the surgical procedure. This is faulty diagnostic reasoning at its worst. Unfortunately, in a medical milieu in which technologic diagnosis is feasible and relatively easy to accomplish, there is a tendency among some physicians to employ tests simply because they are available. If the principles of hypothesis setting and data evaluation enumerated in this text were taken into account, children with recurring abdominal pain characteristic of the psychosocial syndrome would almost never be subjected to such diagnostic and therapeutic procedures.

What we must learn to do is to establish a diagnosis of psychosocial origin of abdominal pain and focus our diagnostic and therapeutic attention on that hypothesis. Unfortunately, many clinicians are untrained and unskilled in this area and find it easier to resort to organic diagnosis and mechanical remedies rather than to expend the time, energy and skill that it takes to approach the logical and highly probable hypothesis correctly.

It is true that in about 5% or less of children presenting with recurrent abdominal pain a detectable organic cause will be present. In his analysis of the data the clinician should be alert to any clues that might indicate the presence of such diseases as are enumerated above. Genitourinary disease is an important component and careful review of urinary symptoms and signs should be made. In addition, those gastrointestinal causes listed above may have specific symptoms or prior history that can serve as valuable clues. For example, if a child has had several bouts of undiagnosed fever in the past and he presents now with abdominal pain, one may logically elevate regional enteritis or urinary tract infection to a higher probability than if the history were negative in the same child. In addition, if the symptoms of recurrent abdominal pain have a consistent pattern in relation to meals, one may suspect intermittent volvulus as a possibility. If the child has had acute episodes of gastroenteritis in the past that were undiagnosed, one may wish to consider chronic infectious or inflammatory disease of the bowel at a higher order of probability than if these symptoms were not present.

In some children with chronic abdominal pain the clinician may wish to employ simple diagnostic procedures, such as urinalysis and examination of the stool for occult blood, as a guide to determination of further investigation. However, if the clinician truly considers this an example of recurrent abdominal pain on a psychosocial basis, undue emphasis should not be given to these screening techniques, and they should be presented to the family in a minor, almost-offhand way. In no case should the patient be made to cling to the finding as critical, nor should there be planted in his mind the idea that further diagnostic studies are indicated, but that you are reluctant to do them. This point cannot be overemphasized because of the frequency of the syndrome and the repetitive practice of escalation of diagnostic tests.

Chapter 17

The Child with Gastrointestinal Bleeding

INTRODUCTION

Bleeding in a child is always a frightening symptom to parents. Educated to the seriousness of this symptom in their own health, they are certain it heralds terrible consequences in their infant or child. Thus, a child with gastrointestinal (GI) bleeding is almost always brought to medical attention immediately, even if the amount of bleeding has been slight.

GI bleeding occurs in two primary forms: vomiting of blood (hematemesis) or blood passed per rectum (frank bleeding or melena). The causes of each type of bleeding differ sufficiently to merit separate consideration.

THE ETIOLOGY OF HEMATEMESIS

Hematemesis, like many other symptoms in pediatrics, has distinct age-related patterns of etiology. Emesis of blood in the newborn includes diseases not considered again throughout life. Likewise, the causes of hematemesis in children differ markedly from those observed in adults. We shall consider the causes of hematemesis in relation to separate age groups.

The Newborn

A common cause of hematemesis shortly after birth is regurgitation of swallowed maternal blood. Varying from a small amount to massive quantities, it is necessary to distinguish this type of hematemesis from other causes originating within the infant.

During the birth process a considerable quantity of maternal blood may be ingested by the infant. Shortly after birth this blood may be vomited, sometimes forcibly. The infant generally appears well, and eventually clears his GI tract of maternal blood.

A relatively simple maneuver will differentiate maternal blood from that of the infant. The infant has fetal hemoglobin which will not react with strong alkali. The addition of 0.25 N sodium hydroxide to the blood will turn a tap water suspension of the bloody specimen to brown-yellow if only adult hemoglobin is present (the Apt test). A pink color results from fetal blood reacting with the sodium hydroxide.

Infants stressed by a variety of diseases may develop ulceration of the upper GI tract. Hematemesis of bright red blood may be the first evidence of such ulceration. Likewise, severe hemorrhagic gastritis may produce the same symptom.

Rare today because of routine vitamin K administration, hemorrhagic disease of the newborn can produce upper GI bleeding. The amount of blood vomited is variable, and if enough is passed through the GI tract, black stools may result. This type of bleeding may be associated with purpuric lesions in the skin or bleeding from the umbilical stump or circumcision site. The disorder is due to vitamin K deficiency, normal in newborn

153

infants, or may be secondary to liver disease or other disorders of the coagulation mechanism.

Although peptic ulceration of the duodenum has been reported in newborn infants, it often is confused with stress ulceration in an infant who has a serious disease, such as bacterial meningitis, sepsis, or other disorders.

Only on rare occasions will infants with congenital anomalies of the GI tract, such as reduplication, Meckel's diverticulum, or intestinal obstructions produce enough bleeding in the newborn period to result in hematemesis.

The Infant and Young Child

Hematemesis in this period of life may be related to coagulation disorders, localized abnormalities in the GI tract, or the child's own blood swallowed from the site of bleeding in the naso-oropharynx. On occasion, ingestion of exogenous toxins, such as iron, may produce a severe hemorrhagic gastritis with hematemesis and shock as primary manifestations. Also, prescribed drugs, such as aspirin, may result in erosions in the upper GI tract with significant bleeding and hematemesis.

Although children with coagulation disorders generally manifest skin bleeding and bleeding at other sites such as the genitourinary tract, on occasion the hematemesis may be a component or the primary manifestation of the bleeding diathesis.

Lesions of the GI tract from the esophagus to the upper small intestine may erode a sufficiently large vessel to produce bright red blood which is then vomited. For example, children with esophageal varices from a variety of causes may have considerable venous bleeding manifest as hematemesis. On occasion, duplications of the GI tract, or even Meckel's diverticulum, may contain gastric mucosa which undergoes peptic ulceration, erosion of a major vessel, and massive quantities of GI blood. It is true that in most instances of this type of blood, melena is the most common manifestation, and hematemesis is rare.

A major cause of vomitus of swallowed blood is nosebleed. The child or parent may be unaware that the nasal mucosa is bleeding,

particularly when the site is posterior. However, most nosebleeds will occur in the anterior portion of the nose, and hematemesis in these circumstances is usually easy to identify, since external bleeding has been evident. Less commonly, the bleeding may be from the oropharynx or of dental origin. Of course, if tonsillectomy or other surgical procedure has occurred, considerable quantities of blood may be swallowed and subsequently vomited.

Hemorrhagic gastritis and ulcerative disease of the upper GI tract can occur as a result of exogenous ingestion of poison or drugs. Most commonly, iron, often ingested by toddlers, or aspirin is the inciting cause. On occasion, ingestions of acids or alkalies may be sufficiently corrosive to produce hematemesis. Children with this type of bleeding almost always have concomitant pain, either from the corrosive action of the ingested material at any point along the upper GI tract or secondary to violent contractions of the stomach and intestine secondary to the contained blood.

The Older Child and Adolescent

Older children and adolescents may have any of the forms of bleeding described for infancy and childhood. In addition, a few children in these age groups may attempt suicide with a variety of compounds which can be corrosive to the upper GI tract. Rarely, in a severely disturbed adolescent, self-mutilation may produce bleeding and swallowing of ingested blood with resultant hematemesis.

Children who have severe vomiting from any cause may develop hematemesis of partially digested blood. This so-called coffee-ground material can vary in quantity from very small amounts to extremely large amounts.

Some children in this age group will have long-standing hepatic disease with resultant portal hypertension, and esophageal varices may have been present for some time. An episode of hematemesis in such an individual should immediately suggest its origin.

On rare occasions in the older child and adolescent, lymphomas or other tumors may erode vessels in the GI tract and produce hematemesis.

THE DIAGNOSTIC APPROACH TO HEMATEMESIS

Of primary concern to the physician who first encounters the patient with hematemesis is the determination of the stability of the cardiovascular system. The vomiting of fresh blood or coffee-ground material simply heralds the problem for the clinician but is not necessarily quantitatively related to the actual degree of internal bleeding or severity of the underlying cause. All of us have seen children who have vomited seemingly small quantities of blood, only to develop shock rapidly because a larger quantity of blood was within the GI tract but not vomited. Likewise, what seems to be enormous quantities of blood may be associated with relatively trivial causes, such as nosebleed and swallowed blood.

The first efforts, then, are directed towards determination of blood pressure, pulse, and respiratory rate. As the clinician moves through other considerations, he will take measures to monitor these parameters continuously in order to develop some idea of the progression of the process. It is wise at this point to establish an intravenous line and withdraw blood for blood typing and cross matching, even if the specimen ultimately is not utilized.

Only when these measures have been taken should the clinician proceed to the search for etiology. Even cursory consideration of the causes should indicate the approach that will be taken. Rapid historical discernment of any preexisting conditions, of prior episodes of bleeding, of other evidence of bleeding, and of other prominent symptoms should be made. Clues obtained from such history should be substantiated by simultaneous physical examination to determine whether a site of bleeding is present in the upper GI and respiratory tract or to determine whether there are extra GI tract sites of bleeding, such as in the skin, eye grounds or urinary tract. The physical examination can then be expanded to search for diseases which might be present in the child and which may have precipitated the episode of bleeding.

If the child is in shock or in impending shock, measures will be taken to counteract that homeostatic disturbance prior to any attempts to stem the flow of blood or identify its origin.

The course that is then followed diagnostically will vary, depending on the clues or lack of them obtained from the history and physical examination. For example, if it has been determined that there is brisk bleeding from the nares or a tooth socket, the clinician may restrict his further diagnostic activities to the placement of a gastric tube and efforts to stem the flow of blood from the local site. If the child has had an opportunity to ingest a corrosive substance, the appropriate emergency maneuvers will be made, depending on the nature of the ingestion. For aspirin and iron it may be critical to remove gastric contents, whereas if the ingestant is an acid or alkali, such maneuvers may lead to perforation and should be avoided.

In almost all instances of significant upper GI bleeding the placement of a tube into the stomach will be of considerable assistance in determining the quantity of blood present and the continuation of blood loss. The nature of the material may also give indirect indication as to the level of GI bleeding. With continual removal of bright red blood from a tube placed in the stomach one may suspect an esophageal or gastric origin, whereas if only coffee-ground material is obtained, the bleeding point may be more distal.

Obviously the diagnostician will be guided, in part, by age-related causes. Bleeding within the first hour of life will prompt an Apt test on the recovered material, whereas such testing would not be performed later in the newborn period or at any point in infancy or childhood. If esophageal varices are strongly suspected based on prior history or on physical examination, an appropriate maneuver will be put into effect to both diagnose and treat the bleeding point. If a coagulopathy is suspected, appropriate specimens will be obtained for coagulation profile to pinpoint the defect and direct therapeutic management.

It is not the purpose of this text to discuss in detail the specific methods whereby each of the diseases above is diagnosed and treated. It is important and pertinent to stress that the initial management of hematemesis varies very little from patient to patient with only a few exceptions. The speed and urgency of specific measures to counteract bleeding, shock, coagulation disorders, etc. are totally dependent on the patient's condition and on the clinical clues derived from the history and physical which suggest probable hypotheses.

RECTAL BLEEDING AND MELENA

In contrast to hematemesis, blood loss per rectum has a great many more causes, including many which are trivial. Despite this, most parents and children will bring rectal bleeding to the attention of the physician immediately, and thus the diagnostician may be confronted with relatively minor amounts of bleeding in an otherwise normal-appearing infant or child. Once again, the child with rectal bleeding will have different causes, in part, dependent on his age. We shall consider these causes in age-related fashion.

The Newborn Infant

The newborn infant who ingests maternal blood may exhibit hematemesis, melena or a combination of both. Blood appearing in the stool may be bright red but more commonly is of a darker color. It will be perceived later than will hematemesis and may not be so quickly associated with the ingestion of maternal blood. All infants who pass blood per rectum in the newborn period should have an Apt test performed on a specimen in order to rule out this possibility.

Likewise, hemorrhagic disease of the newborn, as previously discussed, may result in bleeding in the GI tract at a point where the blood is perceived per rectum rather than in the vomitus. Similarly, any cause of upper GI bleeding may result in the passage of blood through the GI tract and its resultant appearance in the stool. Thus, stress ulcers, acute hemorrhagic gastritis, and other forms of inflammatory and vascular bowel disease may result in rectal bleeding.

In recent years, necrotizing enterocolitis has become a more prominent entity in newborn medicine. The precise etiology of this disease is not known, but one component is vascular insufficiency of a portion of the GI tract. Bleeding may be a prominent feature, and bright red to dark red stools may be observed. The infant is usually sick with vomiting, diarrhea, or both, and roentgenologic examination will often demonstrate air in the walls of the intestine.

Although inflammatory disease of the small and large bowel can occur in the newborn, it is sufficiently rare as not to be a prominent cause of blood in the stools. Mechanical disorders, on the other hand, may manifest during the newborn period, and if vascular compromise or ulceration occurs, the stool may be bloody.

The Infant and Young Child

In young infants a common cause of bright red streaking on the stool or presenting at the anus is related to small fissures developing at the anal outlet. These fissures may appear spontaneously or be related to a constipated character of the stool. The amount of blood is always slight and most often accompanies passage of a stool, frequently streaking the external surface. The infant is otherwise well.

In female infants, particularly in the postnewborn period, the appearance of blood in the diaper or on the perineum may be of vaginal origin and not related to rectal bleeding at all. This phenomenon is related to maternal hormonal withdrawal in the female infant.

A prominent reason for rectal bleeding in young infants and children is gastroenteritis. Bacillary dysentery typically has a component of rectal bleeding, and organisms such as *Shigella* and *Campylobacter* are regularly associated with blood in the stools. On occasion, however, a child with severe viral diarrhea may have small amounts of blood observed in the diarrheal stool. This is often related to a degree of proctitis or anal fissuring as a result of severe diarrhea.

Occult rectal bleeding to frank hemorrhage may result from a variety of lesions involving malformations of the GI tract. Meckel's diverticulum may contain gastric mucosa and ulcerate with minimal to massive amounts of bleeding. The blood may be bright-red to dark-black in character. Likewise, the volvulus may produce rectal bleeding. Differentiation between these conditions is often possible on clinical grounds in that volvulus is almost always associated with crampy abdominal pain, whereas Meckel's diverticulum almost always is painless bleeding.

A highly disputed cause for rectal bleeding is cow's-milk allergy. To most of us there can be little question that in some infants a significant degree of bleeding occurs as a result of exposure to cow's milk. I have personally cared for several infants in whom almost exsanguinating hemorrhage occurred each time cow's milk was introduced into the diet after a milk-free period. Lesser degrees of bleeding are also attributed by many to cow's-milk allergy. Often other symptoms of allergy are manifest in the infant, and other GI symptoms may be present, such as vomiting, diarrhea or loose stools, abdominal bloating, and frank abdominal pain.

A typical syndrome has been described in intussusception. In this condition a portion of the GI tract invaginates within itself, resulting in intermittent abdominal pain associated with the passage of the so-called "currant-jelly" stool. However, intussusception is sufficiently variable in degree and recurrence that minor amounts of bleeding may be present, or the stool may contain frank red blood.

In older children, localized lesions within the GI tract may erode and produce bleeding. Intestinal polyps, various types of hemangiomas and other benign tumors, and malignant tumors may give rise to significant rectal bleeding.

Coagulation disorders at any age may produce variable amounts of blood in the stool.

Toxic ingestions of the type indicated under hematemesis may also produce bloody stools or melena.

Inflammatory disorders of the bowel (regional enteritis, ulcerative colitis) tend to occur in older children and adolescents. However, the first episode may occur in a younger child and may be associated with some rectal bleeding.

Any of the lesions described under hematemesis may also produce a sufficient amount of blood passed through the GI tract, leading to melena. Thus esophagitis, gastritis, peptic ulceration of duodenum, and esophageal varices can be manifest solely as blood passed per rectum or in combination with hematemesis.

The Older Child and Adolescent

Many of the causes discussed in infancy and early childhood obviously equally apply to this age group. In addition, rectal manipulaion, particularly if homosexual, or even simple exploratory activity results in trauma to the mucosa. On occasion, bizarre manipulations (such as objects forced into the rectum) are employed and can result in considerable rectal damage and bleeding.

Although hemorrhoids are rare at any age in childhood, their appearance begins to be noted during adolescence. On occasion, hemorrhoids may bleed and produce symptoms similar to those observed with anal fissure.

THE DIAGNOSTIC APPROACH TO RECTAL BLEEDING AND MELENA

Since a wide variety of causes may result in blood in the stools, and only rarely will the quantity be sufficient to be life-threatening, the clinician generally relies more heavily on history and physical examination to guide him in his ultimate diagnostic pathway.

Obviously age will be important, as outlined above, and certain conditions will be sought almost automatically, given the age of the infant.

A similar homeostatic analysis will be made for the infant with rectal bleeding, although a far larger number of this group will have only minor amounts of blood and no real threat of shock or death.

After rapid initial assessment in this area, the clinician will rapidly proceed to delineate selected characteristics. The quantity of blood and the history of its appearance are very important in distinguishing such minor causes as anal fissure from the potentially more serious precursors. Since there is a wide variety of conditions which can result in rectal bleeding, the clinician will search through the history for the presence of concomitant or preexisting disease, for familial history, for the exact character of the bleeding, and for the possibility that the red material observed was, in fact, blood. Red food coloring, either natural or artificial, can survive passage through the GI tract and result in the appearance of red stools. A history of the ingestion of large quantities of red-colored food, such as beets or materials artificially colored, will be useful. In addition, certain medications, such as ampicillin, are delivered in a red dye-based liquid which also can survive transit. Although history alone will not provide conclusive evidence that this is the cause of the discoloration in the stool, it may lead to prompt testing for blood and elimination of this category of disease.

The physical examination will concentrate on the anus, rectum and abdomen but will also sample for the presence of other disease. It is particularly important to search for bleeding elsewhere in the body, as indicated under hematemesis. The abdominal examination will concentrate on the presence of mass, tenderness, or other signs indicative of an inflammatory or obstructive process. In young infants, particularly those with a small amount of blood, careful examination of the anus may reveal the presence of a fissure. Rectal examination, manually or by means of an infant or child proctoscope, may be extremely useful in identifying inflammatory and traumatic lesions in the distal colon.

The stool content should always be analyzed for blood, even if the material seems obvious. In the neonate one would wish to distinguish maternal from fetal blood, and in older infants and children, to establish that it is indeed blood.

Subsequent laboratory and roentgenologic analysis will be almost totally dependent upon the individual condition or conditions suspected. In both hematemesis and rectal bleeding, judicious use of such modalities as endoscopy and roentgenologic examination of the GI tract is mandatory. It is beyond the scope of this chapter to enumerate the indications for each of these diagnostic approaches. Their application will flow from the initial hypotheses generated and the degree to which they can identify the lesions suspected.

Surgical intervention in either condition is likewise dependent on the specific hypotheses generated, their probability of being present, and confirmatory diagnostic tests, if such are

necessary. For example, in the infant with currant-jelly stools, abdominal pain and a palpable mass, one may strongly suspect intussusception, and diagnostic utilization of the barium enema may also be therapeutic. On the other hand, if the intussusception is identified but is not easily reducible, surgical intervention may be necessary. This is but one example of the progression from initial suspicion through diagnosis and management. Obviously, for individual circumstances the progression may differ and the modalities employed be specific to the disease or condition sought.

Unfortunately, in a given percentage of children, no underlying lesion may be identified despite utilization of all diagnostic modalities. In fact, in rectal bleeding it has been stated that as many as 25% of children will not have a provable cause for their rectal bleeding. It is also true that diagnosis may not be achieved for an initial episode. In one patient in our experience, 2 years passed with multiple episodes of rectal bleeding before a large Meckel's diverticulum was identified and surgically corrected. This infant had several different diagnoses attributed to her rectal bleeding prior to identification of Meckel's diverticulum. This particular lesion can be very difficult to identify, and newer radioisotope localization techniques have been utilized in an effort to reduce the failure rate.

One might argue that in such a serious symptom as GI bleeding, a negative diagnostic assay should culminate in an exploratory laparotomy to provide the diagnosis. It is sobering to know that among the group in which no diagnosis has been reached, exploratory laparotomy has been used. Most pediatric surgeons will indicate that this procedure of external inspection of the GI tract in a child in whom all other diagnostic studies are normal or negative is most often nonproductive. In fact, several consultants with whom I have worked over the years refuse to consider exploratory laparotomy at that juncture in a child's evaluation for precisely this reason.

Chapter 18

The Child Who Fails to Thrive

INTRODUCTION

Of necessity, many weeks or months of an infant's life must lapse before determination is made that he is "failing to thrive." This catchall phrase is commonly used to indicate a failure in weight gain, although stature may also be affected in some infants. This slowly evolving state may be unrecognized in its early stages, or multiple forms of nutritional alteration applied, each of which lead to delay in diagnosis and progressive worsening of the infant's status.

Unfortunately, there are no universally accepted, clear-cut definitions such as "so many grams of unachieved weight in such-and-such" a period of time. Many clinicians will consistently plot the patient's weight, height and head circumference on a growth grid. They begin to become suspicious of failure to thrive if the child deviates from his own apparent path of growth.

Some physicians use the third percentile as a cutoff point for such determination. With deviation below this level from a previous pattern above it, or with consistent weight and height below the third percentile, a presumption of failure to thrive is made. It is clear that some individuals in this latter group are small throughout life without any discernible cause for failure to thrive. This is believed to be on a genetic or constitutional basis and implicit in the chromosomal makeup of the individual. These children will not be further considered, although they do need to be differentiated from the remainder of the group which has a definable cause.

Failure to thrive almost always has psychologic impact on the family. As we shall see, in one instance the psychologic impact may be the antecedent to failure to thrive. However, in all instances, deviation from a family's or society's expectation can result in feelings of guilt, inadequacy or even hostility on the part of the parents and relatives. Depending on the state of development of these emotions, the comprehensive evaluation of such children may be complicated, and false clues followed. Such emotions cloud historical recounting, often resulting in the parent overemphasizing some points in the history and underemphasizing others. In addition, one may find that the informants include a wider circle than with other conditions, and it is not uncommon for grandmother, aunt or some other relative to provide unsolicited history during the course of the investigation. Often these tidbits of historical information are offered in the midst of considerable family controversy and on occasion can lead to enormous confusion as to the actual sequence of events. This phenomenon is mentioned here because accurate historical delineation is important in some forms of failure to thrive. If the physician is deceived by parents on a conscious or unconscious basis, and if he believes such deceit to be true, he may pursue elaborate and unnecessary diagnostic pathways or fail to pursue certain lines of inquiry that might be more productive.

With these facts in mind we shall now consider the causes of failure to thrive.

THE ETIOLOGY OF FAILURE TO THRIVE

There are many reasons children do not continue a normal growth pattern. Display of such a list leads one to believe that a disorganized and seemingly random series of events can terminate in failure to thrive. However, a definite pattern emerges if one groups the causes into some basic underlying mechanisms. First, there is a group of causes related to inadequate intake of calories. Obviously a child will not gain weight or grow in linear length if inadequate nutrients are supplied or accepted.

Second, there is a group of disorders in which growth failure occurs despite adequate caloric intake. More often there is a disproportionate decrease in linear growth compared to weight gain. A large and diverse group of conditions can contribute to such growth failure, including genetic, structural, endocrinologic and related causes. Third, some children fail to thrive on the basis of a central nervous system defect. In some cases this defect is clear-cut and definable, whereas in others it is only suggested by inadequate cerebral growth but no specific definable lesion.

It is in the context of these three general categories of growth failure that we shall enumerate the specific lesions.

Inadequate Intake of Calories or Nutrients

An infant may not receive an appropriate caloric intake based on improper feeding practices, because of a disturbed maternal-infant relationship, or because of a firm cultural belief in a given dietary pattern which deviates from acceptable caloric and nutrient standards. In addition, in a few infants the caloric intake may be sufficient but rejected by the infant or, if accepted, regurgitated. In this latter group, disorders in swallowing, fatigue upon sucking or eating, or various forms of vomiting may be observed.

Many parents are unprepared for the role of nurturer of their infants. In some instances an uneducated, mentally retarded, or inadequately prepared parent will have no concept of normal infant requirements and will either not seek professional instruction or will misinterpret or not understand it, if offered. In such instances the total amount of calories offered to the infant is below that required for normal weight gain and linear growth. In our subsequent analysis we will indicate methods that the clinician may use to detect this type of abnormality.

In some infants even adequate amounts of calories offered are simply not ingested. The infant may experience difficulty in swallowing or sucking based on underlying neuromuscular or structural disease in the esophagus or oropharynx. Sucking and swallowing require an orderly sequence of neuromuscular function with automatic generation of impulses from the central nervous system, coupled later in life with learned responses, such as chewing, to complete the process. Infants who have significant central nervous system disorganization may be unable to suck on a natural or artificial nipple or may be unable to propel ingested fluid or food towards the stomach. Some disturbances in esophageal motility and function of the esophageal-gastric junction limit the infant's capacity to ingest an appropriate quantity of milk or other nutrients or cause such foodstuffs to accumulate in a greatly dilated esophagus. Often the third type of pattern mentioned above will supervene, and vomiting or regurgitation or rumination of ingested food will occur.

In some infants with debilitating cardiopulmonary or chronic infectious disease and other disorders the energy required for feeding is simply not musterable. A typical example is the infant who has incipient congestive heart failure in which the first sign may be inadequate feeding. The infant tires easily during the sucking and swallowing process and will refuse to continue the activity despite apparent hunger and loss of weight. In some infants with chronic infectious diseases, marked apathy towards food, i.e., a combination of anorexia and fatigue, will result in inadequate caloric intake. In some endocrine disorders, (e.g., hypothyroidism) the child will be hypotonic and easily fatigable, and inadequate food intake will result in weight loss or failure to gain weight. Finally, some children who have malabsorptive syndromes resulting ordinarily in adequate intake but incomplete digestion and absorption will also manifest anorexia and fail to thrive.

In abnormal physiologic function and actual obstruction of the gastrointestinal tract, intake may be inadequate, even though the offered food is proper as to volume and caloric content. In such individuals, vomiting or other forms of regurgitation will be obvious, and usually provide adequate clues to the underlying process. However, in a few such individuals the loss of ingested food will be minimal with each feeding, and inadequate intake will only be suspected in retrospect, when the child fails to gain weight. In addition to abnormalities in structure and function, chronic metabolic conditions, such as diabetes, persistent acidosis, or specific metabolic disorders, may be associated with vomiting and inadequate intake. Subtle and slow increases in intracranial pressure, such as occur with hydrocephalus or subdural hematomas, may result in persistent and protracted vomiting leading to failure to gain weight.

In a small percentage of disordered maternal-infant relationships the amount of food offered the infant may be inadequate in relation to his needs. In many such instances the actual amount of food is adequate but the lack of appropriate emotional interaction may result in inadequate utilization. Which of the two forms is operative in a given circumstance will require certain diagnostic observations which will be detailed later.

Growing in frequency is the number of young parents who have opted to pursue a life-style which differs from that of the majority of American parents. As part of this alternative approach to living, the parents often adopt different and sometimes bizarre feeding methods for their infants. Vegetarian diets, a variety of "natural" food regimens, diets which eliminate milk or dairy products, and many other unique forms of diet are found in such subcultures. The result in the infant may be an inadequate caloric intake in general, or specific nutrient deficiencies which impair growth and orderly development. In many infants the process is a slow one and only evident after months of exposure to the abnormal diet. This is particularly true if the diet offers enough calories but is deficient in protein or some other nutrient.

Infants Who Fail to Thrive despite Adequate Intake of Calories

There are two major causes of inadequate growth despite exposure to an adequate diet. The largest group of disorders is related to malabsorption in which nutrients pass through the gastrointestinal tract and are excreted in the stool. A second category, actually part of the first but distinguishable because no specific defect can be diagnosed, is the group of constitutional causes. In this category, adequate, or even enormous, quantities of calories may be ingested, but the individual remains thin and small, presumably on the basis of some genetic or chromosomal predisposition which results in either decreased absorption or decreased utilization of absorbed foodstuffs.

Malabsorptive syndromes are extremely variable in specific mechanism. The malabsorption may be part of a diffuse process, such as cystic fibrosis, or may be very specific to a given enzyme system in the gastrointestinal tract. Complete enumeration of all malabsorptive syndromes is beyond the scope of this text. However, the commonest causes include cystic fibrosis, pancreatic insufficiency, celiac disease, tropical and nontropical sprue, immunologic deficiency, chronic gastrointestinal infections, lymphatic abnormalities of the gastrointestinal tract, monosaccharidase and disaccharidase deficiencies, and a variety of other discrete disorders. Malabsorption may be across a broad spectrum of nutrients, as occurs in chronic inflammatory disease, or may be confined to a specific component such as carbohydrate or lipid.

In many of these infants the appetite is voracious, and reconstruction of the diet leads to unbelievable amounts of ingested food. In almost all instances the stool pattern will be abnormal, the specific characteristics of which are dependent upon the type of absorption. The child may have watery diarrhea or loose stools if the absorptive defect is generalized, may have bulky, foul-smelling, fat-filled stools if the absorptive defect is for lipids, and may have diarrhea with a very irritating stool which "burns" the perineum if carbohydrate intolerance is the cause. In the latter instance, the stool contains a high acid content as the malabsorbed carbohydrate is converted to corresponding organic acids.

Disorders of Growth Associated with Central Nervous System Abnormalities

Structural, functional or chronic inflammatory disease of the brain may be associated with failure to thrive. Although ultimately this type of lesion will fall in either the first or second category enumerated above, it is deserving of separate consideration, since the diagnostic focus will not be on intake or the lack of it but on the underlying cerebral cause. The specific disease or condition may be identifiable. For example, a large porencephalic cyst, chronic subdural hematomas, or progressive hydrocephalus may be present. On the other hand, the defect may be more subtle and not identifiable as a specific structural abnormality. In fact, in a proportion of infants the only clue to cerebral origin of the failure to thrive is inadequate growth of the brain as manifest by a lag in head circumference. In many such infants, all available diagnostic procedures simply point to a small brain with no specific structural abnormality. In addition, certain forms of maternal deprivation, which will be detailed later, may also result in a cerebral type of failure to thrive, the precise mechanistic nature of which is undiscernible.

Maternal-Infant Deprivation Syndromes

I would like to separate from the discussion above a particular subset of infants who fail to thrive based on lack of adequate emotional interaction between the caretaker, usually the mother, and the infant. It is clear from Henry Silver's study of large numbers of such infants that a variety of subsets may be discernible. In some cases it is simply a parent who is unprepared for that role who treats the infant with indifference, largely out of ignorance and/or their own flat emotional affect. This type of disturbance is particularly seen in the young teenager, often a single parent, who is attempting to rear a child at a period in life when neither expectation nor maturity permits an adequate emotional interaction with the infant.

A separate subset is found among mothers who have serious organic or functional disorders. The mother who is severely mentally retarded or who has a severely impairing psychotic state may fail to care for an infant adequately, secondary to these conditions.

Another subset is the group of parents more commonly associated with child abuse. In such individuals a pattern of hostility and neglect has been present in their own lives, and they rear their own children similarly. In the most "benign" form of child abuse, simple neglect of the infant with inadequate feeding and inadequate attention to maternal-infant interaction may be present. In other forms the neglect and failure to thrive is only one component in which actual physical or sexual abuse also occurs. In the latter group attention is often focused on the identification and repair of the physical injury, and only secondarily is it appreciated that the infant is also failing to thrive on the basis of inadequate nutrition or inadequate emotional support.

In the final subset, no clear-cut and obvious pattern is immediately discernible that falls in any of the above categories. However, upon observation of the maternal-infant interaction, it is clear that adequate "chemistry" does not occur between mother and infant. In these circumstances the mother will treat the infant as an object rather than as another person, and the feeding becomes mechanical and eventually is abandoned in a personal sense to the propping of the bottle or the delegation to some third party. There is little or no play activity between parent and infant, and the infant is often left alone in the crib without any human contact for long periods of time. Such parents may not display classic psychotic symptoms or overt evidence of abusive feelings or behavior towards the infant. They appear to be simply indifferent and to lack any qualities of human warmth that most of us associate as a natural phenomenon in maternal-infant interactions.

Regardless of the exact mode, the effect on the infant is the same. He becomes apathetic and unresponsive to his environment and often will develop repetitive automatic behaviors, seemingly in an effort to provide some stimulation which is lacking otherwise in his life. There is little interest in sucking or feeding, almost as if the infant comes to regard it as mechanical an act as does the caretaker. On occasion such infants will appear to be apprehensive upon the approach of any other human into their immediate environment or, on the other hand, will be extremely apathetic and indifferent to such approaches.

On occasion, even the well-intentioned mother will encounter an infant who, for reasons that are as yet unclear, does not participate in maternal efforts at interaction. Whether this is a subtle neurologic deficit or some other constitutional or genetic trait is unclear. The effect on the parent occasionally is one of lack of reward for the efforts that are made, and indifference, apathy or even outright hostility may result. In some situations the combination of an unresponsive infant and a potentially abusive or indifferent parent reinforces the negative interaction and leads to an almost-complete separation between the two members of the maternal-infant unit. Some individuals regard infantile autism as an extreme example of this form of indifferent interaction. In autism the infant may develop into an individual who is totally devoid of responsiveness to any animate objects in the environment. The focus appears to be upon inanimate objects and behaviors that do not depend upon interpersonal reactions.

THE DIAGNOSTIC APPROACH TO THE INFANT WHO FAILS TO THRIVE

It has become my firm belief that in most instances in which significant failure to thrive has been detected, a period of in-hospital observation is essential. There are two major reasons for such removal of the infant from the natural environment. The first is to afford the diagnostician an opportunity to observe both the infant alone and the infant in relation to the mother under controlled circumstances. In this endeavor the clinician should utilize one or more ancillary medical personnel to assist in the evaluation. In many units, one or a few nurses have been well trained in making such observations and are assigned to the maternal-infant pair in question to record in extended fashion the observable interactions. The second reason is to afford an opportunity to provide an adequate diet by a third party, usually a nurse or aide, and to record the infant's response.

As part of this early phase of observation the diagnostician is also afforded an opportunity to explore in detail all historical elements that might lead to placing the child in one of the etiologic groups mentioned above. A history of dietary intake is mandatory, as is the exact feeding practices that are employed. In addition, some estimation must be made of the usual maternal-infant interaction during and between feedings. A careful history of all of the caretakers who participate in the child's care should be obtained, and their exact role in relation to feeding delineated.

Additional historical information of use in such infants is the presence or absence of vomiting, the precise nature of sucking and swallowing, the precise sequence of diet from the preparation of foodstuffs to the actual offering to the child, delineation of a host of symptoms that may be related to any of the categories listed above, including the frequency and nature of the stool, the presence of symptoms in other systems, such as the respiratory tract or central nervous system, evidence of urinary tract or other anomalous findings, and the emotional responsiveness of the infant in a variety of situations.

Anticipating that most thorough histories will tend to place the child in one of the major categories above, the physical examination will, in part, be directed by such categorization. For example, if it has been clearly established by history that the dietary intake has been inadequate, the usual pediatric physical examination will suffice. If, on the other hand, the diet offered has been adequate but the infant has failed to thrive, attention may be more carefully paid to the neurologic examination and to examination of the abdomen.

It should be clear at this point that if one considers the largest number of children who fail to thrive, the history and physical will be unrewarding except for the actual feeding practice, the amount of food offered and taken, and some hints as to maternal-infant interaction. In these instances it is wisest to proceed in very cautious and conservative fashion in relation to subsequent diagnostic testing. In fact, only very simple tests should be employed initially, such as a complete blood count, urinalysis, examination of the stool for occult blood, and by culture, and little else. Rather, the focus should be on observation—observation of the infant during the usual feeding practice by the principle caretaker. In conjunction with this, in several feedings the usual caretaker should be substituted for the experienced nurse mentioned above who attempts to feed the infant in a "motherly" fashion. This is actually a diagnostic test in which the infant's sucking, swallowing and emotional interaction to the feeding process are carefully observed and recorded. Of necessity, this period of observation should be of sufficient length to establish clearly both the natural caretaker's and the hospital caretaker's observations. It would be inappropriate to make a judgement after only one or two feeding episodes, since the change from the home environment to the hospital environment may in itself be initially disturbing to the pair. Although no firm time guidelines can be provided, it is my opinion that several days should go by of such observations before any further judgements are made. If, in fact, deficiency in feeding practice or maternal-infant interaction is apparent during this period, it should be extended for as long as several weeks in order to add the next essential component, which is detection of the infant's weight response to alterations in either the feeding practice or the social interaction. It has been our observation, as well as that of others, that in both disordered feeding practice and inadequate maternal stimulation, weight gain may be seen in the hospital, and an awakening of the infant's interest in his human surroundings will be observable. This valuable diagnostic test can then direct future efforts at counseling and correction of the basic underlying interpersonal disorder or mechanics and avoid the necessity for expensive and unnecessary diagnostic procedures.

If, on the other hand, the initial period of observation, or anything in the initial history and physical examination, suggests that one of the mechanical or functional causes within the infant are responsible for failure to thrive, the appropriate course can be pursued. If vomiting or regurgitation is a major component, morphologic studies and functional studies of the upper gastrointestinal tract will be necessary. These can be accomplished by appropriate radiographic procedures, as well as by such techniques as placing a probe in the esophagus looking for regurgitation of gastric acid, or even by endoscopy. It is obviously impossible in a text of this sort to track every single diagnostic pathway that will be undertaken. The individual conditions and the degree to which they are suspected will assist the clinician in ordering the appropriate diagnostic tests in sequence.

In malabsorptive defects great attention must be payed to both the content of what is ingested and the specific content of the stool. Measurement of fat in the stool and various tests to detect specific components, such as the disaccharides, may be necessary in specific instances. If the defect is felt to be a more generalized one, such as cystic fibrosis, attention should be payed to diagnosis of that basic condition, with sweat electrolytes coupled with analysis of stool content.

In central nervous system disorders it may be necessary to employ radiographic and other techniques to detect mass lesions or abnormalities in cerebral spinal fluid flow.

If there has been significant vomiting, one may wish to pay attention to homeostatic measures as well as the specific diagnostic tests to uncover the cause of the vomiting. It will be necessary to assess serum proteins and electrolyte concentrations and, in some instances, to search for metabolic derangement in other systems.

If a metabolic abnormality is suspected, appropriate diagnostic tests aimed at the established hypotheses should be undertaken.

At this juncture it is imperative to reiterate and reemphasize that a willy-nilly differential diagnostic approach to the child with failure to thrive is *most inappropriate*. Perhaps nowhere else in pediatric practice is there as great a tendency to list all the possible causes of failure to thrive and to undertake their simultaneous evaluation immediately upon entry to the hospital. In these circumstances, infants have been subjected to a bewildering variety of radiographic, metabolic, stool and serum examinations in such rapid sequence as to result in inadequate nutrition simply because the infant was never on the unit or was being held without feedings prior to specific tests during the initial period. We have encountered such infants who have continued to fail to thrive in a most critical acute way because of the multiple and sequential tests, most of which were unnecessary.

As pointed out elsewhere in this volume, differential diagnosis has its place in the practice of medicine. It is seldom useful in infants with failure to thrive. The process has been slow, and the defect is a generalized one without any specific life-threatening components at the moment. At least this is true for the vast majority of infants who present with failure to gain weight or grow adequately. In a few instances, specific abnormalities may be present which do, in fact, warrant rapid and complete delineation, but these are in such a minority that to employ such techniques across the whole spectrum of this disorder is inappropriate.

Among inexperienced diagnosticians it is tempting to plunge ahead with the differential diagnostic approach. This is generated out of insecurity or because of the symmetry in diagnosis that is perceived by considering the etiologic classifications above. It is extremely attractive to the inexperienced diagnostician to be able to employ specific tests, both of a screening and definitive nature, in each of the areas above. This tendency must be avoided for the reasons listed.

The aftermath of initial diagnostic efforts is also a clinical problem-solving process. If the clinician has discerned one of the maternal deprivation syndromes as being operative in a specific infant, the approach is one of solving that particular problem. Why has the interaction gone awry? To answer this type of secondary hypothesis question, the clinician often must employ not only his own skills but those of a variety of consultants, including the social worker, the public health nurse, the psychologist and, on occasion, the psychiatrist. These consultative diagnostic

encounters should be viewed in no different fashion from a radiographic or laboratory sampling for organic disease. The data should be carefully considered in the light of the hypotheses generated, and an attempt should be made to determine if the hypothesis has been substantiated or rejected, or something in between.

Unfortunately in this area it is all too common for the clinician to be enamored with the initial steps in diagnosis and in the establishment of the primary hypothesis. Thereafter, the diagnostic process loses its "glamour," and the patient is relegated to other professionals for continuous care or continuation of the diagnostic process. It is my feeling that this is a grievous error and not consistent with total care of the maternal-infant combination.

A similar sort of delegation of diagnostic responsibility occurs in the organic sphere. Children who have their failure to thrive on the basis of endocrinopathies or metabolic or gastrointestinal disease may well be shunted off to a specialist, who then pursues that area in detail but often ignores other aspects of the infant's well-being. Since failure to thrive occurs at a period in life when total general pediatric care must be extended to the infant, it is imperative that a primary care physician be involved at all stages. This is a logical extension of the clinical problem-solving process, albeit more comprehensive and more thorough and requiring a slower and more continuous process than does the acute resolution of the infant's initial diagnostic riddle.

On occasion we have seen infants who have failed to thrive and have had an adequate diagnosis established initially, only to have the symptoms persist or recur after an initial period of adjustment. In almost all instances this has been related to inadequate continuation of the problem-solving process and to indifference, neglect or delegation of the secondary hypotheses resolution. I use this example to emphasize this point particularly, although it is true of many of the other problems discussed in this text. Although it may seem a bit philosophical and even "preachy" to dwell on this subject, I find that the opportunity is most affordable in considering failure to thrive rather than in some of the more acute problems whose resolution occupies a smaller span of time.

It is also important in this context to understand the long-term implications of early infant malnutrition. We are coming to recognize, as long-term follow-up studies are completed, that there are critical periods in development during which malnutrition exerts an adverse affect on cognitive, emotional and other aspects of development. Infants malnourished early in life may sustain a prolonged deficit in cerebral function or in emotional reactivity which will require continuous evaluation and rehabilitative efforts to the limits of the child's capacity. This continuous problem-solving process is essential if maximal function is to be achieved by the patient.

It also brings us full cycle to the initial discussion at the heading of this chapter in which the diagnosis of failure to thrive may be long delayed. Armed now with the knowledge that infant malnutrition has potentially serious consequences for ultimate brain development, it becomes even more imperative that such infants be identified early in the course of their malnurtured pattern and that diagnostic steps be undertaken. One measure that will assist in this regard is the employment of some continuous diagnostic scheme to measure the rate of growth and the rate of development in the infant. It is beyond the scope of this text to indicate the various measures that are available, but employment of some growth grid and some developmental screening device, such as the Denver Developmental Scale, can be of immeasurable aid in such evaluation. Further, the physician is urged not to ignore early signs of failure to thrive and not to employ dietary change in an attempt to reverse the process. It is not uncommon for months to pass before the infant is subjected to diagnostic scrutiny. Occasionally during this interval, multiple formula changes and introduction of a variety of foodstuffs have occurred concomitant with continual failure to thrive of the infant. I believe that this prolongation and delay in diagnosis is directly attributable to the lack of application of the principles of problem solving to the earliest manifestations. The clinician who first confronts an infant who is falling below standards for his age is tempted to succumb to the easy hypothesis that something is wrong with the formula that is being fed the infant. In most instances this turns out not to be true, but despite this known fact the practice continues and lingers. One purpose of knowledge of the problem-solving process is to bring it to bear at an appropriate interval in a given patient's problem. Nowhere is that more evident than in the child who fails to thrive.

Chapter 19

The Child with a Rash of Infectious Origin

INTRODUCTION

It would be presumptuous in a textbook such as this to attempt definitive diagnosis of childhood rashes. To do so would require extensive description of a multitude of diseases plus adequate illustration, since the Chinese were correct when they asserted that one picture is worth 10,000 words. However, the child with an infectious rash does present an opportunity for reasonable analysis of an area that particularly lends itself to sequential diagnosis.

Therefore, the reader should not treat this chapter as a do-all and end-all for the diagnosis of infectious disorders with a skin rash. Rather, he should utilize it as a model of diagnostic reasoning in which a combination of factors are brought to bear to reach acceptable hypotheses.

GENERAL CONSIDERATIONS IN THE DIAGNOSIS OF INFECTIOUS DISEASES WITH RASH

In any child who presents with a rash as a major or sole complaint, a number of factors must be taken into consideration in reaching a diagnosis.

Obviously, the first consideration is the actual appearance of the rash and a description of each of its characteristics. Second, the onset and progression of both the rash and its accompanying disease manifestations are critical. Third, the past history of infectious diseases and, in some instances, of immunizations received will be helpful. Lastly, simple diagnostic tests employed to extend the data base are also useful. In the latter circumstance we are not referring to specific diagnostic tests that are addressing a major hypothesis. Rather, it should be viewed as a search to add bits of data, often necessary in order to generate an appropriate hypothesis.

Let us first consider in more detail the rash itself. One of the commonest failings in diagnostic efforts in this area is for the clinician to gloss over the rash and treat it with only a cursory attempt at definition. This can be a grievous error, since the actual character of the rash may in itself be most revealing of the underlying diagnosis. Rashes are not infinite in variety; in fact, they can be separated conveniently into morphologic groups. Many such groupings have been proposed and utilized by various diagnosticians. I will utilize my own schema, which will fit into our ultimate diagnostic differentiation.

Infectious rashes may be divided into (1) macular eruptions, (2) maculopapular eruptions, (3) papulovasicular eruptions, (4) urticarial eruptions, (5) petechial eruptions, (6) erythema multiforme and similar rashes, (7) eczematous dermatitides, and (8) combinations. Extensive descriptions of each of these characteristics can be found in textbooks of infectious diseases and dermatology. For our purposes we will consider macular eruptions as flat, nonpalpable lesions. Maculopapular eruptions will have this characteristic plus small, raised solid lesions, whereas papulo-vasicular eruptions include eruptions in which there are small, raised solid lesions plus fluid-filled vesicles.

There are variants in each of these categories in relation to size. I will include nodular lesions under maculopapular eruptions and will include bullous lesions under papulovesicular eruptions. Nodules and bullae differ respectively from papules and vesicles only in size.

Urticarial lesions include a wheal, usually associated with considerable itching. Petechial eruptions may take any of the previous forms but contain extravasated blood.

Erythema multiforme refers to a specific type of lesion in which the so-called iris or bull's-eye lesions are predominant. That is, there is an expanding erythematous lesion which clears centrally. On occasion, erythema multiforme may actually have a bullous component and is referred to as erythema multiforme bullosum. One variant of the latter is called Stevens-Johnson syndrome, which involves both mucosal membranes and the skin.

Finally, a few infectious diseases will demonstrate variable components, including several of the above categories.

In addition to these morphologic differentiations, rashes will also differ in color, in discreteness, in density, in shape and in distribution. Each of these is important in defining individual disease entities. For example, the lesion of measles can be described as "a maculopapular, confluent, generalized erythematous eruption which begins at the hairline extending caudad generally over a period of 3 days." As one can see from such a description, it is specific. One does not refer to the measles rash as a red rash all over the body. This type of description is of no use in differentiation and should be avoided at all costs.

The onset and progression of rash is important in relation both to itself and to other symptoms which may be present. One must carefully ascertain whether the rash appeared first or occurred during the course of other infectious symptoms. Following delineation of onset, one should then describe the progression of the rash thus far. Did a generalized rash appear simultaneously in all parts of the body, or did it progress, as in the description of measles above, over a period of time, to become generalized from a focal origin? Also important during this historical search is the concomitant progression of other symptomatology. One can extend the description of measles above as follows: "This child developed the sudden onset of fever to 104° F associated with coryza, followed in a few hours by photophobia, which has become intense in the past 2 days. A marked, dry, barking cough has been observed in the same time period. The child has become anorectic with easy fatigability and marked irritability. After 2 days of these symptoms the rash described above appeared and progressed as described." As one can see from this description, a very specific syndrome has been elicited with whose onset, association with other symptomatology, and progression a definitive pattern has emerged. When one adds the description of the rash to such a characteristic onset, one is two thirds of the way towards a specific diagnosis. Given such a description on the telephone, a diagnostician may already place measles as his number one choice, with a high degree of probability of being correct.

In addition to accurate description of the rash and its associated symptomatology, one must also search out past history in the child as well as in contacts. In this case, one attempts to exclude one-time diseases, such as measles, since their occurrence precludes the current episode from being that disease. Of course, great care must be taken in this area, since many rashy illnesses are misdiagnosed, by either the patient or physician, and the same care in description of disease must be exercised in obtaining a past history as is exercised with the current episode.

In addition, one wishes to elicit an accurate history of immunizations in the past in order to exclude or include certain diagnoses. Further, a history of similar disease at an appropriate interval may suggest that the child currently has the same disease as seen in siblings, classmates or other contacts. Thus, in the child with measles, one might elicit the following history: "This child has had no measles immunization nor history of any previous rashy illness compatible with measles. Two weeks ago a cousin who stayed at this child's house had a rashy illness similar in all respects to this child's. The other child also did not have a history of prior measles immunization." In such an instance as that described for measles, one can almost be 100% certain that he is dealing with measles simply by elicitation of an appropriate history. Subsequent physical examination, as will be described later, will then be confirmatory, given such a classic pattern.

Not many diagnostic tests will add to our data base in infectious diseases. Commonly employed are the total white blood cell count and differential. In this instance the clinician may take a puzzling rash and attempt to decide whether a bacterial or viral disease is present. The usual caveats are necessary in extrapolating such results to diagnosis. Not all viral infections have low total white blood cell counts with predominance of lymphocytes, and not all bacterial diseases are associated with an elevated white blood cell count and a shift towards the polymorphonuclear series.

In some instances, examination of the lesion itself may yield a clue as to its origin. For example, in certain vesicular lesions, scraping the base may reveal giant cells which are characteristic of certain deoxyribonucleic acid viruses (herpes simplex and varicella-zoster). In certain rashes a specific group of organisms may be suspected by detection of a characteristic morphologic appearance with special stains, e.g., yeast particles in fungal dermatitis and gram-positive cocci in impetiginous lesions.

On occasion the use of ancillary diagnostic tests, such as fluorescence under Wood's lamp examination, may suggest certain of the superficial fungi.

The physical examination will follow the same format as for history. One wishes now to obtain as accurate a description of the rash that is currently present as is possible, classifying it according to some simple schema, such as the one given above, with care taken to be precise and complete. The child should be totally unclothed, or alternatively, the entire body examined sequentially if modesty is a factor. Under no circumstances should a diagnosis of rashy illness be made unless all parts of the body have been examined. In

circumstances in which immediate diagnosis is impossible, sequential physical examinations over time may be required, which will then add some direct observational knowledge of the progression of the rash and its characteristic evolution. Of course, a physical examination will also include data on other manifestations of infections in organs and systems other than the skin.

DIAGNOSTIC REASONING IN INFECTIOUS RASHES

Under "General Considerations" I suggested that a complete historical and physical examination delineation be made of the lesion. At the other end of the spectrum, the physician must be familiar with the common infectious diseases and their characteristic descriptions, onset, progression and association with other symptomatology. In addition, he must be aware of simple laboratory tests which add to his data. The diagnostic process then becomes one of pattern recognition alluded to previously in an earlier chapter. What the physician does is to match the characteristics observed in the patient against the typical characteristics of a variety of infectious diseases. Depending on the degree of symmetry, he establishes hypotheses with varying probability. In the example of measles given above, knowledge of the characteristic pattern of that disease matched against the description given yields a very high probability for measles.

Certain infectious diseases will only produce a macular eruption. For example, certain staphylococcal diseases associated with an erythrodermic toxin will produce a flat or macular erythematous eruption. Many virus infections will result in dilatation of superficial skin vessels, leading to a blotchy erythematous rash which is often generalized. Roseola will produce a generalized, very small (just a few millimeters in diameter) erythematous macular eruption. The lesions of secondary syphilis are also generalized, macular and erythematous. Certain forms of leprosy may result in colorless atrophic areas of skin which are macular. Macules also occur in the superficial fungal infections and in pityriasis rosea. In these latter diseases the macules may scale early, leading to a characteristic appearance.

The list of papulovesicular eruptions is large and includes most of the major childhood contagious diseases. Measles, German measles or rubella, scarlet fever, certain forms of meningococcemia, many of the rickettsial infections, and a variety of viral infections, including cytomegalovirus, enterovirus, Epstein-Barr virus, and Kawasaki's syndrome, are all associated with maculopapular eruptions. In addition, some forms of staphylococcal infection, meningococcemia and toxoplasmosis also will have maculopapular eruptions. These rashes are not all alike, although on occasion they may mimic one another. For example, measles will produce a generalized, maculopapular, confluent erythematous eruption that is reasonably characteristic in appearance. On the other hand, rubella may resemble the rash of measles or may be much milder, less confluent and less generalized, and more transient. Scarlet fever produces a sunburned appearance to the eye and a sandpaper feel to the rash on physical examination, revealing its papular characteristic added to its macular component, which is visualized. In meningococcemia the maculopapular eruption may be sparse and widely distributed and may occur prior to the characteristic petechial nature of this disease. Enteroviral infections, on the other hand, may resemble any of the diseases above or may include generalized maculopapular eruptions which do not fit into any of those categories.

Papulovesicular eruptions include the various lesions of the herpes group, including herpes simplex, varicella and zoster eruptions. In the past, vaccinia and smallpox occurred with greater frequency than they do today and also were manifest by papules and vesicles. One of the rickettsial diseases produces typical vesicular lesions; rickettsial pox is a disease rarely seen with this characteristic eruption. The Coxsackie A and B viruses may be associated with characteristic vesicles, and occasionally papules, on the skin and mucous membranes. Molluscum contagiosum has an extremely characteristic papulonodular component with a vesicular core. Children with eczema may become infected with deoxyribonucleic acid viruses, such as herpes and vaccinia, and a characteristic papulovesicular eruption results. Staphylococcal impetigo characteristically begins as small vesicles with a purulent content.

Urticarial eruptions caused by infectious agents are uncommon. Some of the enteroviruses will produce an urticarial component. On occasion, acute infectious diseases may be associated with urticaria as they progress. Atypical measles, a form of disease seen in previous recipients of killed measles virus vaccine, often has an urticarial component in combination with other types of eruption.

Petechial rashes may be observed characteristically in meningococcemia in which the rash is produced by local capillary blockage by the organisms. These eruptions contain the organisms, which can be identified on histologic examination.

Petechiae also occur in a wide variety of enteroviral infections and may be a component of any of the communicable diseases, such as measles, if thrombocytopenia is present. Hemorrhagic varicella and, in the past, hemorrhagic smallpox also produce petechial lesions as well as frank extravasation into more characteristic vesicular components. Infectious mononucleosis (Epstein-Barr virus infection) also may be associated with a petechial rash. Many of the rickettsial infections will have petechiae as one component. Severe gram-negative infections associated with disseminated intravascular coagulation may be associated with bleeding into the skin.

Erythema multiforme may accompany or follow a number of acute infections. It is particularly prevalent in acute coccidioidomycosis. It is also a major component of the recently described Kawasaki's syndrome (mucocutaneous lymph node syndrome). In addition, patients with *Mycoplasma pneumoniae* infections will often have an erythema multiforme eruption of the bullosum variety. In the latter circumstance the mucosa is also involved.

Eczematous eruptions are uncommon in pediatrics as a consequence of infectious diseases. They are occasionally seen with superficial fungi, such as *Candida albicans* dermatitis.

Combinations of the above eruptions may be seen most commonly in enteroviral infections but can occur in atypical forms of any of the diseases. Combinations are particularly seen in immunosuppressed or immunodeficient individuals in which the characteristic pattern may fail to appear owing to a faulty immunologic response.

Such a listing obviously does not include all infectious diseases with a dermatologic component, nor do all diseases neatly fit into their particular category in every patient. Frustrating as this may be, it simply represents truth and must be taken into consideration in atypical, difficult cases.

Armed with an accurate description of the present illness in the patient and some knowledge of his past history, as well as similar episodes in contacts, the clinician will attempt to match these characteristics with the known characteristics of the commonest infectious diseases. This pattern recognition is also assisted by knowledge of the characteristic symptomatology for that disease in organ systems other than the skin. As illustrated in the measles example above, the characteristic rash occurs in the setting in which cough, coryza, fever and photophobia progress in classic fashion. On examination, apart from the characteristic eruption, an intense conjunctivitis and oropharyngeal nonspecific inflammatory response is also observed which completes pattern recognition. In measles there is also pathognomonic Koplik's spots— small white plaques a few millimeters in diameter occurring on the buccal mucosa. This is one of the few pathognomonic signs in medicine, and ordinarily the clinician is not aided by such specificity.

In learning about infectious diseases with rash and in committing such patterns to memory the diagnostician is well advised to consider the following categorizations: existence of a prodrome, type of onset, characteristic progression of symptoms and sequence of manifestations, and laboratory aids.

Measles may be contrasted with rubella in that the former has a 3- or 4-day prodrome, as described above, whereas rubella ordinarily presents with the rash and little or no prior symptoms. The classic prodromal illness is illustrated by roseola or exanthema subitum. This disease occurring in young infants has a 3- or 4-day period of intense fever with no other manifestations. The rash appears, often as a transient phenomenon, as the fever reaches its peak on the third day or at any time thereafter. This pattern is characteristic enough to suggest this diagnosis in an otherwise well-appearing child with fever for 3 days. Variable prodromes for the other maculopapular eruptions can only be learned by studying the individual diseases.

Similarly, for each of the other categories of illness a prodrome may or may not be present and may or may not be characteristic in its description.

Such characteristics as onset and progression, with particular attention to the sequence with which symptoms appear, is also of importance. For example, the classic progression from prodrome to rash to healing that occurs in measles has been alluded to above. Few other diseases will resemble, even in a superficial way, this characteristic progression. Thus, measles recognition is relatively simple, since most patients will exhibit each of the characteristic features, and the features themselves are sufficiently unvarying to allow the diagnostician to hold a given pattern in his mind. On the other hand, the enteroviral illnesses are produced by a hundred or more viruses with extreme variability in patterns. A few are characteristic, such as the papulovesicular eruptions with Coxsackie agents and certain of the exanthems associated with the enteroviruses. Again, this text cannot pretend to offer you complete analysis of each of these syndromes, but one would be hard pressed to make a specific diagnosis unless one was familiar with the major categories.

SUMMARY

In the final analysis, diagnosis of rashy illnesses depends on astute observation and history taking to delineate the exact characteristics of the rash that are presented by the patient. At the same time the clinician will observe the epidemiologic and clinical setting in which the rash occurs, and if diagnosis is not immediately apparent by appropriate pattern recognition, a period of observation may yield sufficient data as to progression and evolution to enable the clinician to reach a correct diagnosis.

If the clinician cannot label a specific infectious rash, he will move to specific diagnosis. Employment of the laboratory tests to be discussed is not the same as the screening tests alluded to earlier which add to the data base. These tests are specific in nature as to etiologic agent and are employed in narrow or wide fashion, depending on the degree of probability of a specific group of agents being present.

The clinician has at his disposal a variety of means for testing his established hypotheses. If he suspects a specific infectious disease, the search for that agent will be determined by the available diagnostic tests. For example, if measles is suspect, the clinician may either attempt to isolate measles virus or simply demonstrate a rise in specific antibody around the illness. Suggestive evidence for the presence of measles may be obtained by smears of the nasal mucosa looking for characteristic giant cells, called Warthin-Finkeldey cells.

In other circumstances the clinician may suspect that he is dealing with a bacterial, viral or fungal infection but cannot be more specific than that. In these cases, material will be taken from the patient, either from the skin rash itself or from inflammatory exudate elsewhere, and appropriate histologic examination or cultures undertaken. In rare instances, with severe disease, a simultaneous search may be made for a number of different pathogens, since a characteristic pattern does not emerge or is not recognizable.

This final stage in diagnosis will complete the pattern recognition response.

Chapter 20

Detailed Analysis of a Single Child with Pharyngitis

INTRODUCTION

In this chapter I am going to "talk" you through the diagnostic steps involved in a single child with pharyngitis. In contrast to previous chapters, I will not offer a separate account of etiology of pharyngitis but will integrate this information into the actual analysis of the child's illness.

The narrative is in great detail—even obvious steps have been included. The instance is real, the reconstruction as accurate as I can make it. This child's illness has served as an example of the diagnostic method for more than a decade. She is unusual, but the value of recounting her illness *is not* in her diagnosis, but in the step by step process by which it was reached. Along the way we will learn a great deal about a great many illnesses, but, of most importance, we will trace the diagnostic reasoning employed by her physicians.

Her diagnosis is unimportant (in terms of the educational lesson). I will repeat this at the end of the exercise in order to emphasize it.

JOY'S ILLNESS—PART 1

Joy is a 5½-year-old white female living in Laramie, Wyoming. She was in good health until the onset of her illness, when she complained of a sore throat and of feeling hot. Her temperature was 104° F, and her parents sought medical care for her. Her family physician observed a markedly reddened pharynx, cervical lymphadenopathy which was tender, and a temperature of 104.5° F. In addition, he felt she looked "toxic," as evidenced by her flushed facies, disturbed countenance and moderate irritability.

Analysis Thus Far

Her physician believed Joy to be infected with Group A beta-hemolytic streptococci (GABS). He reached this conclusion because of her sudden onset of fever, the complaint of sore throat, the finding of tonsillopharyngitis, and anterior cervical adenitis. In addition, he was aware that in that particular geographic region, GABS was prevalent, and many additional cases had been seen in the recent past.

His reasoning was of the pattern recognition type. On the one hand, he knew that GABS was characterized by fever, sore throat, "toxicity" (i.e., systemic symptoms of lassitude, fatigue, malaise, irritability, anorexia and, occasionally, even vomiting), evidence of erythematous to exudative inflammatory changes in the pharynx and tonsils, and cervical adenitis. In some children a scarlatiniform rash and/or palatal petechiae may also be observed.

On the other hand, he observed in Joy a cluster of compatible symptoms and signs, none of which were inconsistent with GABS. Please note that she did not have all possible signs or symptoms associated with GABS, but neither did she have any which could not be attributed to this infection.

This is an example of sequential diagnosis, as outlined in an earlier chapter. The clinician does not consider a complete differential diagnosis of pharyngitis at this point, since it would be both unnecessary and wasteful of his time and effort, and conceivably of the patient's time and money, should he choose to pursue unlikely possibilities. The critical question confronting him is how compatible is this child's symptom complex with that which he has stored in his own memory bank for GABS. The answer is obvious: highly compatible. He also knows that clinical diagnosis of GABS is not totally reliable. Even children who manifest a 100% correlation of the so-called classic symptoms of GABS may, in fact, have another etiologic agent present. We will further consider this point at a subsequent time in our analysis. For the present it is important to recognize that the only serious diagnosis entertained by the clinician is streptococcal pharyngitis. If he were forced to assign a probability to the correctness of this hypothesis in this particular child, the level would probably be at 70 to 75% certainty. This figure is based upon several published series in which compatible clinical symptomatology was compared to final diagnosis reached on microbiologic grounds.

Having accepted this major hypothesis, the clinician is now prepared to act. Although a variety of choices is available to the clinician, this particular practitioner chose simultaneously to obtain a throat culture for beta-hemolytic streptococci and to treat the child as if his certainty was higher than 75%. He administered intramuscular penicillin in the office, followed by oral therapy to be continued at least until the results of the culture were known.

In this case his test is very specific. His hypothesis is GABS, and the test is designed to ask the laboratory simply whether or not streptococci of the appropriate type are present. The test is reasonably sensitive. At that time in Wyoming a streptococcal screening program utilized the growth of bacteria (obtained from a throat swab) in broth and the identification of streptococci, if present, by fluorescent antibody methods. With an appropriately obtained specimen the yield of this particular technique is 95% or higher;

that is, in 100 cases of streptococcal disease proved by other more elaborate methods, the particular technique utilized will identify 95 or more instances. There were no false positives with this technique as then employed.

The choice of antibiotic has also been based upon the clinical reasoning of many investigators in which the objective is to rid the child of the streptococci in order to prevent rheumatic fever. Such therapy must be continued for at least 10 days if streptococci are present in order to insure that all organisms are destroyed and an aberrant immunologic response does not occur. Thus the clinician in this particular case instituted his therapy based on the high probability of his being correct but with the fact that he could alter or stop the oral administration of antibiotics should his original hypothesis not be sustained.

JOY'S ILLNESS—PART 2

Forty-eight hours after receiving the intramuscular penicillin, Joy's symptoms had continued unabated, and her physician admitted her to the hospital because, in addition to the original findings, vomiting, respiratory distress and delirium had been observed at home. Her physical examination was unchanged except that she now had marked exudate in her tonsillopharyngea! area, her fever was of the spiking type, often reaching 105 to 106° F daily, and her cervical adenitis had increased in severity.

Analysis at This Point

At this point the clinician was uncertain as to the correctness of his original diagnosis. The original throat culture had not yielded any streptococci, but he was aware of the up to 5% incidence of false negative test results by the technique employed. Therefore, he did not wish to abandon his original hypothesis completely but added to it the possibility that the child was suffering from one of several forms of viral pharyngitis. He added these possiblities to his list of hypotheses because she had not responded to penicillin, her throat culture was negative for streptococci, and he knew that the next largest group of organisms which produced streptococcal pharyngitis was certain of the ribonucleic acid and deoxyribonucleic acid viruses. He was particularly aware that infectious mononucleosis, caused by Epstein-Barr virus, was very frequent in mimicking streptococcal pharyngitis.

At this point he repeated the throat culture, this time submitting it to the routine microbiology laboratory in the hospital for more complete identification of organisms that might be present. He also obtained a white blood cell count and differential in the hope that this would help to differentiate between a bacterial infection (in which case he hoped to see an increased white count with a shift to polymorphonuclear elements) and viral pharyngitis (in which case he expected to see a low white blood cell count with a shift toward the lymphocytic series). In addition, he wished to have the laboratory examine the peripheral blood smear for the presence of atypical lymphocytes, a finding which is characteristic in the early stages of infectious mononucleosis.

Thus, with a minimum of laboratory tests, he undertook to reconfirm or reject his initial hypothesis (that of GABS) and to screen for the presence of viral pharyngitis, which is the next logical category.

At the same time, he was disturbed about the effect the illness was having on the child's homeostasis and undertook to hydrate her by intravenous fluids and to attempt to control the temperature by antipyretics.

JOY'S ILLNESS—PART 3

Joy remained in the hospital in Wyoming for 6 full days. During this period the symptomatic therapeutic measures reduced but did not eliminate the fever and a tendency towards delirium at the height of fever. She became reasonably well hydrated, and the physician had little fear that further imbalance would occur as long as he was controlling her fluid and electrolyte intake by intravenous administration.

Her physical findings did not change significantly except to exacerbate in quantity. Her cervical adenitis became even more marked, and her tonsillopharyngitis developed an even greater exudative appearance.

Despite her complaint of respiratory distress, no physical findings were detected in the lung, and the physician did not order a chest X-ray.

Her laboratory studies revealed a pure growth of *Candida albicans*, an ubiquitous fungus, from her throat culture; a total white blood cell count of 10,200 with 50% polymorphonuclear leukocytes and 50% lymphocytes, none of which were atypical in character; and a heterophile.

The clinician continued penicillin therapy to which he added sulfisoxazole, but neither antimicrobial appeared to influence the course of her illness.

Further Analysis

At this point in her diagnosis her clinician became increasingly concerned that his original hypotheses were incorrect. He now felt reasonably certain that she did not suffer from streptococcal pharyngitis, and he did not believe that infectious mononucleosis was present, although the evidence for or against this diagnosis was scant. He also worried about the persistence of her symptoms, seemingly unabated, which suggested to him that a more serious infectious process, or even a noninfectious one, was responsible for her illness. However, he had reached the limits of his diagnostic knowledge in this group of disorders and decided that he needed consultative advice, and turned to a large academic medical center.

When Joy's symptoms were described to the consultant, he, too, could not readily explain the child's symptomatology. The consultant agreed to accept the child in transfer in the hope that a more detailed examination and assessment might yield the correct diagnosis.

Prior to transfer the referring physician had obtained several blood cultures which were still incubating in the laboratory. He also had obtained a heterophile titer, since he felt he did not have an adequate test for the presence or absence of mononucleosis. However, he did not wish to await the results of these tests, since he felt the child's clinical condition warranted further assessment. Accordingly, the child was transferred to the academic medical center.

JOY'S ILLNESS—PART 4

On admission to the university hospital, Joy's history was substantiated as had been obtained previously. A complete physical examination revealed the following positive findings: (1) a temperature of 105° F; (2) marked constant apprehension and anxiety; (3) vesiculopustular lesions of the lip and mucocutaneous junction; (4) shallow ulcerations (three in number) of the oral mucosa and palate; (5) necrotic yellow-gray membranous tonsillopharyngitis; and (6) large tender anterior and posterior cervical lymphadenopathy. Specifically sought but not found were skin rash, abnormal pulmonary findings, hepatosplenomegaly, and generalized lymphadenopathy.

Continued Analysis

At this point the consultant was faced with a child who had been ill for almost 9 days with symptoms that were slightly progressive since the initial onset and which had changed only slightly in character. Vesicular lesions of the mucocutaneous junction and shallow ulcerations in the oropharynx had not been described previously. At this point he was aware of the negative blood cultures at the other institution, of the two throat cultures which were negative for streptococci, and of the negative tests for infectious mononucleosis. Even cursory consideration of the child's clinical circumstances suggested serious disease and increased the need for a complete differential diagnostic approach. The reason this mode of diagnosis was attempted should be clear from the detailed discussions in the early chapters of this volume.

The consultant briefly considered the possibility that beta-hemolytic streptococcal disease was, in fact, present but had not been adequately diagnosed. This seemed an untenable conclusion in view of the two negative throat cultures and the pattern of this particular infection, which was inconsistent with streptococcal disease which tends to improve after 3 or 4 days irrespective of whether specific therapy has been employed. Thus the initially generated hypothesis by the primary care physician was rejected thoroughly at this stage. It is important to point out that reconsideration of that initial hypothesis was essential in order that it not be overlooked as a possibility, however remote. The consultant recognized that should he have begun with this as a new problem, he may or may not have considered streptococcal disease, which could have worked to the patient's disadvantage.

Viral pharyngitis, even infectious mononucleosis, could not be effectively ruled out despite the negative blood smear and heterophile test thus far. The consultant argued that the initial rise in atypical lymphocytes may have been missed on original smear, and it may have been too early to detect heterophile antibody levels in the serum. At the time this child was seen, there were not the rapid screening techniques available for mononucleosis, and this is the reason they are not reported in the protocol.

In addition to viral causes, the consultant began to consider less frequent, and even rare, causes of oropharyngeal exudative infections. The recovery of *C. albicans* raised the possibility that this organism was pathogenic in this child. However, *C. albicans* almost never produces primary pharyngitis unless the individual is immunodeficient or has a lymphatic malignancy. The consultant also recognized that the child had been treated with antibiotics for almost 6 days from the inception of the illness and that the recovery of *C. albicans* may simply have been related to eradication of normal throat flora by the antibiotic, to the possible virus infection that might be present, or to a combination of both. Nevertheless, *Candida* pharyngitis was retained as a hypothesis that was possible, even though of low probability at this juncture.

If this child did not have a viral or fungal cause for the oropharyngeal infection, were there other bacteria apart from the beta-hemolytic streptococcus which could produce this type of disease? The consultant considered the following list of bacteria, each of which will be discussed separately: *Corynebacterium diphtheriae*; *Neisseria gonorrhoeae*; *Staphylococcus aureus*; *Streptococcus pneumoniae*; and *Mycobacterium tuberculosis*. Of these, only diphtheria and gonococcal infection seemed likely, since the throat cultures had not grown the staphylococcus or pneumococcus, which only rarely produce exudative tonsillopharyngitis and then only in immunodeficient or immunocompromised individuals. Diphtheria or gonococcal disease might have been present and not detected by routine blood cultures and therefore remained possibilities to which no probability could be ascribed at present. *M. tuberculosis* is an extremely rare cause of tonsillar exudate, and in general this is the so-called "cold" type; that is, the inflammation is chronic and indolent and not associated with massive acute inflammation. In addition, the tonsillar lesion tends to be unilateral, and there usually is a history of milk ingested from infected animals.

Other extremely rare causes of pharyngeal infection include some of the zoonoses, particularly infection with *Pasteurella tularensis.*

Primary noninfectious causes of tonsillar and pharyngeal inflammation are agranulocytosis and lymphatic leukemia. However, in these lesions the pharyngitis is generally more discreet, with shaggy, even "dirty" ulceration and exudation. The consultant recognized that at least one blood count had not revealed a paucity of granulocytes, nor were any abnormalities described in the lymphocytes observed.

Armed with this rather-thorough differential diagnosis, the consultant then addressed the sequence in which diagnosis might be accomplished. The child was obviously ill and much sicker than the consultant had appreciated when he discussed her with the primary physician prior to transfer. Her previously reported respiratory distress and delirium appeared to be present, particularly at points when the temperature rose above 104° F, and there was concern for her central nervous system integrity as well as for her capacity to sustain enough energy should the process continue without a diagnosis or specific treatment.

One additional consideration at this point was an assessment of her homeostatic disturbance. She had been receiving intravenous fluids for some days now, and the prolonged fever and rapid respiratory rate may have contributed to aberrations in her serum electrolytes, fluid balance and oxygenation.

As a result, the initial sequence involved a rapid assessment of her fluid and electrolyte balance, blood gases and renal function. As these were within normal limits, her maintenance fluid therapy, adjusted for her fever, was continued.

The next order of business was to define her infectious process further to be certain it was limited to the oropharynx. The hypotheses here were that she might have a more generalized viral or bacterial infection with a primary focus in the oropharynx. Cultures of blood, examination of cerebrospinal fluid, a chest X-ray, and urinalysis and urine culture were obtained in an effort to delineate the anatomic extent of her infection.

Parallel with homeostatic and anatomic diagnoses, specific etiologic diagnosis was undertaken. Since it was rapidly determined that her urine, spinal fluid and chest X-ray were all normal, focus again centered on the differential diagnostic list enumerated above. It was felt that diphtheria was most urgent to eliminate or establish quickly, and that sampling for the other major categories might also be accomplished. A smear was obtained for fluorescent antibody determination for *C. diphtheriae*, and a culture for the same organism was established. It appeared unlikely that diphtheria was present in view of the extreme toxicity and in view of the extreme inflammatory response and the lack of specific neuromuscular or cardiovascular toxicity, both of which are features of diphtheria. Nevertheless, these diagnostic procedures were undertaken in the event an atypical presentation was occurring in this girl. It was anticipated this would be a low-yield procedure, and there was sufficient clinical evidence against the diagnosis of diphtheria that no specific antitoxin therapy was initiated.

Cultures of the pharynx were also obtained for viral, fungal and bacterial isolation attempts. Also, the urine and spinal fluid previously obtained and rectal swabs were submitted to the virus laboratory for analysis. It was anticipated that several days to several weeks might pass before any of these cultures would be positive, and hence viral etiology would only be entertained if all searches for bacterial and other causes were negative.

A tuberculin skin test was applied despite the negative chest X-ray and despite a lack of an adequate history at that point. This diagnostic maneuver was attempted despite the conviction of the consultant that it would be of extremely low yield. The clinical manifestations were not consistent with oropharyngeal tuberculosis, which as a result of bovine organisms was exceedingly rare, and the child's pharyngeal state might yield a negative test even if tuberculosis were present. Cultures were obtained and initiated for mycobacterial isolation in the event that all diagnostic tests, including viral, were negative, and if any other clues occurred in the meantime to suggest tuberculosis. Again, this was felt to be a low-yield procedure, but this was one potentially treatable disease which, if present, should be detected.

The possibility that infectious mononucleosis was responsible for this child's syndrome remained uppermost in the consultant's mind. While he recognized that there were some manifestations (oral ulceration, vesicular lesions on the lip) which were not consistent with this diagnosis, and there were signs that the child lacked (no splenomegaly, no generalized adenopathy) and that at least two previous screening tests had been negative, it still appeared to him at this point that the diagnosis had not been adequately excluded. This may be an example of a persistent hypothesis that is not justified on clinical grounds but is retained nevertheless. In fact, in retrospect, it is apparent that the consultant clung to this particular diagnosis far beyond the statistical probability that it was present. Nevertheless, as this was his reasoning at the time, additional studies were undertaken to establish its presence or absence. Repeat white blood cell counts with careful search of the peripheral blood smear were performed, and another heterophile test was ordered. Both were negative for any evidence of infectious mononucleosis.

At this juncture most of the diagnoses in the differential listed above had been entertained. Tests were underway or had been achieved to establish or rule out the individual etiologic agents. Two full days had elapsed, and the child's condition worsened slightly during this interval but was essentially unchanged.

At this juncture the consultant decided to re-review the entire clinical course, the differential diagnoses, and the diagnostic approach thus far. The child's case history was presented to a small group of colleagues, including the entire team responsible for her care, plus several experienced clinicians and infectious disease experts. At the conclusion of the presentation and discussion it was decided that all but the most remote possibilities had been considered, and that these now should be entertained. In addition, it was suggested that the bone marrow be examined and that immunologic capacity be assessed. Although the consultant and his colleagues agreed that there was little or no evidence for the presence of either an immunodeficiency or lymphatic malignancy, the child was sufficiently atypical, and the diagnostic tests carried thus far so unrewarding, that even diagnoses of most remote probability should be entertained and the simplest procedure to establish their absence or presence be carried out. In the ensuing 2 days, bone marrow examination and multiple blood cultures were obtained, the throat culture was repeated, and a reassessment was made of her homeostasis.

All throat cultures revealed pure growth of *C. albicans*, and all other tests, including the blood cultures, were negative.

During this 2-day interval, Cliff Hoyle, a junior medical student assigned to the patient, and the consultant sat down to rediscuss the proceedings of the conference and to re-review her record. From consideration of the differential diagnosis it was clear that a number of historical bits of information had either been cursorily examined, or specific questions had not been directed in areas of potentially low yield. As a result, Mr. Hoyle took the parents aside and, together with the consultant, re-reviewed the entire history, including the span of time 1 month prior to the onset of her illness.

It must be pointed out that this reinquiry was now a highly directed one, based on the hypotheses that had been generated, including those of extremely remote possibility, of rare occurrence, and atypical presentation. This was not simply a repetition of the initial historical search, but one that was carefully designed to elicit specific information from the family.

As a result of this directed inquiry, and keeping in mind the diagnoses listed above, the following facts were discovered: The family lived in a large, well-kept house trailer close to an urban center in Wyoming, although in a quite rural setting. A large pasture adjoined the trailer and was grazed by both horses and cattle. The family kept a short-haired dog and a duckling, both of which were in good health, as had been previously ascertained. There was no evidence of rabbit or other animal habitat in or around the housing. However, the family recalled an amusing tale about the family dog, who was usually an inept hunter. She had continually attempted to catch a large wild rabbit in the adjoining pasture, always without success. In fact, the family recalled that this provided many evenings of entertainment, as their dog appeared to be chasing the same rabbit. About 3 weeks prior to Joy's illness the rabbit disappeared, and it was believed that the previously inept dog had captured it.

In addition, the week prior to the onset of her illness Joy had visited a rural area in Oklahoma, a fact that was previously known. What was not appreciated was that this was her grandmother's farm, and during that excursion she drank raw milk, bathed and played in a known polluted stream, and was discovered to have a tick on her scalp which had been removed just prior to her return home.

These epidemiologic facts suggested to Mr. Hoyle and the consultant that the zoonoses and tuberculosis did have to be seriously considered. It was well known that *P. tularensis,* the causative agent of tularemia, could produce an oropharyngeal form of the disease following ingestion of food or water contaminated with the organism. In addition, tularemia has been transmitted by tick bite, and it was known that this child had had such an episode. It is of interest that the family volunteered none of the information when asked about animal exposure, travel and other infectious contact until specific questions were asked based on the known characteristics of the diseases and the differential diagnosis.

In addition to tularemia, which was made more likely by the child's history, oropharyngeal tuberculosis also had to be considered because of the ingestion of raw milk. However, the interval was exceedingly short, and this diagnosis still appeared unlikely on clinical grounds as well.

With this substantiation of possible tularemia exposure, this hypothesis was raised to one of much higher probability than it had previously occupied. As a result, specific tularemia agglutinins were measured with appropriate controls, and it was discovered that her titer was high and ultimately rose to a level of 1:320. Specific chemotherapy was instituted with intramuscular streptomycin, and the child experienced rapid defervescence with complete and total resolution of the oropharyngeal signs. She was returned to normal health on discharge and continued well thereafter.

FINAL ANALYSIS

I cautioned the reader at the beginning of this chapter that the diagnosis was relatively unimportant. The consultant has not seen another case of this form of tularemia since this child appeared. Of course, the diagnosis was important to this particular child, but it has no value in itself for our considerations here.

What is critical is the sequence of diagnostic reasoning that occurred in the case of this young lady from the inception of her illness to achievement of the correct diagnosis.

We saw original sequential diagnosis with disease of high probability considered initially, appropriate tests carried out, and the child's course followed.

It soon became apparent that the original high-probability diagnosis was not present, and a second order diagnosis, following the usual progression and sequential diagnosis, was then entertained. However, even this diagnosis could not be sustained, and the child's continuing illness appeared to be threatening to her body integrity. At this point we saw the utilization of limit setting by the primary care physician, who recognized that he could not proceed further, and the use of consultation as one means of handling this dilemma.

At the consultant level we saw the need for the change of diagnostic style from that of sequential reasoning to complete differential diagnosis. We understand that this change in style was dictated by the child's worsening condition and frightening disease.

We were exposed to one error in the application of the diagnostic reasoning process, that of persisting with a diagnosis beyond the point at which it should be abandoned. In this regard it is of interest to note how the consultant ignored incompatible signs or decreased their significance in order to sustain an hypothesis that he was reluctant to release.

We then saw a reasonably orderly approach to the multiple diagnostic possibilities, including a sequence of diagnostic tests which was designed to yield diseases which were both detectable and treatable. We also observed the utilization of screening tests for disorders of very low probability, and long-term diagnostic planning by use of such techniques as culture to establish the diagnoses which were thought to be of lower probability but which would require some time (e.g., tuberculosis).

We then observed the reassessment of the differential diagnosis at a point in the child's course when the diagnosis was unclear and laboratory tests inconclusive. By reaffirmation of the original differential diagnosis, two diagnostic pathways resulted. The first included examination for diseases which were thought to be only very remote possibilities and which required more invasive procedures for their detection. The second was reinquiry seeking more data, now directed by the generated hypotheses. And, finally, we saw how this process yielded information which converted a rare disorder of low probability to one of much higher probability in this child, and saw the diagnosis established and confirmed, and the illness treated satisfactorily.

Bibliography

Books*

Elstein, AS, Schulman, LS, and Sprafka, SA: *Medical Problem Solving: An Analysis of Clinical Reasoning.* Harvard University Press, Cambridge, MA, 1978.

    A result of a major research project in the Office of Medical Education Research and Development at Michigan State University, this text attempts to dissect the clinical problem-solving process scientifically and to apply some of the findings to medical education.

Tumulty, PA: *The Effective Clinician.* Saunders, Philadelphia, 1973.

    Divided into four sections, this text combines exploration of clinical communication with issues of management and differential diagnosis in internal medicine. Specific patient-oriented problems are dissected by Dr. Tumulty.

Feinstein, AR: *Clinical Judgment.* Krieger, Huntington, NY, 1967.

    An "old" classic which thoroughly explores a scientific, partially mathematic and statistical approach to problem solving. Rich in detail and the author's experience and wisdom.

Wickelgren, WA: *How to Solve Problems.* Freeman, San Francisco, 1974.

    A delightful paperback volume which considers theory and practice with stratagems for solving problems in general. Heavily influenced by experimental psychology.

Lusted, LB: *Introduction to Medical Decision Making.* Thomas, Springfield, IL, 1968.

    Heavy emphasis on Baye's theorem and its applicability to medical diagnosis. Lots of discussion of statistical concepts and of decision trees. Dissects the problem-solving process and points to human errors. Very sophisticated text, heavily referenced.

Barnoon, S, and Wolfe, H: *Measuring the Effectiveness of Medical Decisions—An Operations Research Approach.* Thomas, Springfield, IL, 1972.

---

* Comments are those of the author.

Sophisticated statistical and theoretic discussions of medical diagnosis and decision making. Emphasis on method of measurement of effectiveness.

Murphy, EA: *The Logic of Medicine.* Johns Hopkins University Press, Baltimore, 1976.

    Intended as a text for first year medical students, this volume covers theory and application of clinical thinking with heavy emphasis on a concept of medicine and on statistical "truth" versus other notions.

Wulff, HR: *Rational Diagnosis and Treatment.* Blackwell Scientific Publications, Oxford, England, 1976.

    A discourse on scientific thinking in clinical medicine. The author dissects the problem-solving process and also includes therapeutic decision making. This text often delves into the actual reasoning process in a specific instance in an attempt to enlighten the reader and to avoid the "mystery" of decision making.

Lipp, MR: *Respectful Treatment.* The human side of medical care. Harper & Row, New York, 1977.

    An "old" text by modern standards, this volume is not about problem solving per se, but about the hazards of treating people as objects. There is much of use to students and residents in this slim volume with a great deal of down-to-earth practical advice.

Journals

    These citations are highly selected and are only of relatively recent origin. For readers who wish to delve more deeply, each is referenced, and older literature can be retrieved in this fashion.

Lintors, EW, and Neelon, FA: The case for bedside rounds. *N Engl J Med* 303:1230, 1980.

McGaghie, WC: Medical problem-solving: A reanalysis. *J Med Educ* 55:912, 1980.

Bosk, CL: Occupational rituals in patient management. *N Engl J Med* 303:71, 1980.

Eichna, LW: Medical school education 1975–79, a student's perspective. *N Engl J Med* 303:727, 1980.

Blois, MS: Clinical judgment and computers. *N Engl J Med* 303:192, 1980.

Thomas, L: On artificial intelligence. *N Engl J Med* 302:506, 1980.

Larkin, J, McDermott, J, Simon, DP, and Simon, HA: Expert and novice performance in solving physics problems. *Science* 208:1335, 1980.

McDonald, CJ, Wilson, GA, and McCabe, GP: Physician response to computer reminders. *JAMA* 244:1579, 1980.

Collins, GF, Cassie, JM, and Daggett, CJ: The role of the attending physician in clinical training. *J Med Educ* 53:429, 1978.

Sisson, JC: Negligence at the bedside: Academic malpractice. *Univ Michigan Med Center J* 42:145, 1976.